Leading a Charmed Life

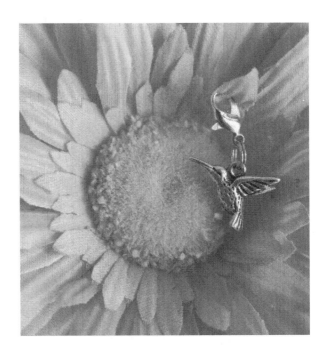

D1534068

Leading a Charmed Life:
My Journey Through Cancer Treatment

Copyright © 2013 by Gayle Bittinger

Photography by Brandie Bracy

Printed in the United States of America

ISBN-13: 978-1493755387

Leading a Charmed Life

My Journey Through Cancer Treatment

Gayle Bittinger

This book is dedicated to John, my husband of 30 years. He is the companion of my heart, my life, and my world.

Acknowledgements

What started as my thoughts written down in some spiral notebooks has become this book because of the many people who love and support me. I want to thank everyone who chose charms for me to write about, including Katie, John, Alex, Marlene, Heather, Hanane, LaLani, Robbie, Laurie K., Tess, my mom, Margaret P., Beth, Dr. Evans, Margaret D., Bobbi, Dr. Rado, Jessica, Jean, Lois, Carleen, and Emily. Your choices and reasons behind those choices inspired me more than you know.

I also want to thank Jean, Heather, Margaret P., Tess, Margaret D., Kimmy, my mom, and John for reading my book in its various drafts and offering suggestions for improvement. I am also grateful to my friend LaLani, who is an English teacher at Mt. Baker High School. She got out the red pen and retaught me the many, many things I'd forgotten from my high school English classes. This book is so much easier to read because of her. In addition, I want to thank Brandie— neighbor, friend, and talented photographer. The pictures she took for this project are better than anything I could have imagined.

My children, Katie and Alex, get a special thanks. Their love and encouragement (and occasional nudging) helped me make this book a reality and not just a dream.

And a big hug and thank you to my husband, John. Your belief in me helped me to believe in myself and what I had to share with others. I couldn't have done it without you.

Introduction

The idea for this journal came to me in March 2011. I had been diagnosed with inflammatory breast cancer five months earlier and had just finished twelve weeks of chemotherapy followed by a bilateral mastectomy. I was looking at eighteen more weeks of chemo, a summer of radiation treatments, and a year of biotherapy infusions, and I had a choice to make. I could let fear and anxiety rule the day, or I could decide that laughter truly was the best medicine and find ways to keep a positive attitude.

I chose the positive attitude. Not a sappy, Pollyanna sort of positive attitude, but instead a determination to find the humor in all of this, to laugh, to focus on what was going right, to enjoy the moment I have right now instead of worrying about a future I could not control. If I wanted to keep up that positive energy, I knew I was going to need a way to count down the next 52 weeks. I felt like a young child 60 minutes into a long car trip asking, "Are we there yet?" So, after considering a variety of options, I decided to start a journal and a charm necklace. Each week I would add a new charm to my necklace and write about it in my journal, letting that charm inspire me to look at my breast cancer experience from a unique perspective.

As the weeks passed, I asked family, friends, and healthcare providers to choose charms for my necklace. Their choices often surprised me, and their reasons for choosing them, if they told me, always touched my heart. And I quickly came to the realization that I am Leading a Charmed Life. Not an easy life, not a trouble-free life, but a life filled with love and surprises, celebrations and joy. What began as a way for me to cope turned into a way for me to reflect and rejoice. This is my story. It is my journey, a record of my thoughts, feelings, and connections made over 52 remarkable weeks. It is my offering to all who walk this journey. May you know in your heart and soul that you do not walk alone.

Table of Contents

Pink Heart

Week 1

This charm was chosen by me.
Why? The heart reminds me of the outpouring of
love my family and I have received. The color
pink stands for breast cancer.

"Write your worries in sand. Carve your blessings in
stone." —Author Unknown

I'm back at the infusion suite at Columbia Basin Hematology
and Oncology in Kennewick, Washington. I've survived six treatments
of the nastiest stuff on earth and a bilateral mastectomy. Now I'm
getting ready to start eighteen more weeks of chemotherapy followed
by seven weeks of radiation, accompanied by a year's worth of
Herceptin infusions topped off with a risk-reducing complete
hysterectomy. Whew. I'm exhausted just thinking about everything
that's ahead of me, which is why I'm learning to take things one day at
a time, learning to trust my journey. I'm discovering that my role in all
of this (appointments, tests, treatments, procedures, uncertainty) is to
trust that I am where I am meant to be, doing what I am meant to be
doing, which is so much easier to do when my worries are scribbled in
sand and my blessings are etched into stone.

According to the National Cancer Institute, one in eight
women will be diagnosed with breast cancer during her lifetime. Never
in a million years did I think I would be one of the ones. I always
hoped I wouldn't be one of the ones, and every October, when all of
the pink stuff came out, I was always thankful I wasn't one of the ones.
But now I am. And it's not as awful as I imagined it would be. It's not
something I'd choose—who would? But it has been an unexpected

source of so many blessings of love, affirmation, assistance, support, friendship, and faith. I don't believe that God chose this for me, but every day I see God working in my life through my experience with breast cancer. I see God in the love of family and friends, in the many ways people have reached out to my family and me, and in the wonderful care I've received from my many healthcare providers.

I am working hard to take care of myself, to allow healing and wholeness to settle in my soul and take root. I want to fill my heart with the blessings of life so that there is no room for anxiety or worry or stress. Ordinary worries are just that—ordinary. The healing, the blessings, the love are what I experience when I look outside the ordinary. Does it really matter if my schedule or, let's face it, my plan for the way my life would go, is messed up? No. Those are the worries I must write in the sand, the worries that disappear with the wind or the waves. What matters are my many blessings waiting to be carved in stone, the ones that stand strong through good weather and bad, through happy times and sad.

The past five months have changed everything for me. I understand what it means to live in the moment. When I think of all that has happened, I realize that it's time for me to get out my chisel and start carving a tablet of love and thanksgiving. It's time for me to let go of the worries and to let the blessings of light and love be the center of my life.

Infinity
Week 2

This charm was chosen by my daughter, Katie.
Why? "It reminds me of a Mobius strip because
things aren't always as they seem, and there's
more than one way to look at life."

Things that are infinite...

the blessings of family and friends
the love my husband and I share
my love for my children
the beauty of a sunset
God's love and grace
memories
gratitude
faith
hope
trust

Things that are finite...

breast cancer
mouth sores
hair loss
breasts
doctors' appointments
chemotherapy
Herceptin infusions
anxiety
worry
time

When I was diagnosed with cancer, my whole world changed. Appointments, tests, surgeries, and treatments loomed ahead of me, seemingly forever. It helped to remember that while many things stretched out into infinity, cancer was not one of them.

It is so easy to concentrate on the finite—on the things I can no longer do, the things I no longer have. But the things that are finite are also the things that are transitory. They are, by definition, the things that do not last. What is infinite is what matters. What is infinite is what touches my heart, speaks to my soul, nourishes my spirit.

When you hold the infinite in your heart,

You understand that you are

Infinitely blessed,

Infinitely safe,

Infinitely loved.

—Gayle Bittinger

Hope

This charm was chosen by me.
Why? Hope is the story I want to tell.

"You live inside the story you tell." —Marilyn Grey

I am at a teachers' leadership conference this week with my husband, John. Well, John is helping put on the conference, and I am enjoying a change of scenery in a beautiful room overlooking the Columbia River and Portland, Oregon. During the conference, I had the opportunity to attend the keynote session with teacher and motivational speaker Marilyn Grey. Marilyn was funny and inspiring. Her core message was, "You live inside the story you tell." Those seven words touched my soul. They made me realize that the facts, the data about what happened, are just that: facts and data. How I interpret the facts and what they mean depends on me and the story I tell about them.

So how do I live inside the story of a cancer diagnosis? At first, it seemed liked the start of a sad and scary tale, filled with worry and stress. It felt like stepping into a strange new world where everyone spoke a foreign language, using words like carcinoma, pathology, biopsy, radiation therapy, chemotherapy, infusions, surgery. The worst part was when I realized that all of those words were describing what was happening to me! Suddenly, this sad and scary tale felt like a B horror movie. There were tears and fears, anxiety and sleepless nights, anger and frustration. I felt helpless and hopeless. And living inside a story like this was miserable.

And while it's challenging to tell the story of a cancer diagnosis in a way that gives me hope, that's what I want to do. The uncertainties and worries, the stress of leaving behind all that is comfortable and familiar make for a depressing story—if that's all I see. The better story, the one I want to tell, looks beyond the sad and scary details to find the blessings. This is the story that sees the miracles around me.

My story starts with family and friends who are walking with me on this journey, holding me up with love and support, help and prayers. They are the reason I can tell a story worth living. The next chapter features dedicated medical professionals working diligently to pinpoint the precise pathology of my breast cancer so I can receive the very best treatment.

There is a chapter about miracles: the miracle of being healthy enough for timely chemotherapy and surgery; the miracle of friends and family sending cards and letters in such a way that my mailbox was filled with personal greetings every day for more than two months; the miracle of learning to take each moment as it comes, enjoying it just the way it is.

This is a story I am still writing. Once I was diagnosed with cancer, my life changed forever. Once I was diagnosed with cancer, I had a chance to choose the kind of story I would tell. And I choose to tell a story of love and faith and hope because I know... "I live inside the story I tell."

Sea Star

This charm was chosen by my husband, John.
Why? "It matters to this one."

The Story of the Sea Star
"As I walked along the seashore this young boy greeted
me. He was tossing stranded sea stars back to the deep
blue sea. I said, 'Tell me why you bother, why do you
waste your time this way? There's a million stranded sea
stars, does it matter anyway?' And he said, 'It matters to
this one. It deserves a chance to grow. It matters to this
one. I can't save them all, I know, but it matters to this
one, I'll return it to the sea. It matters to this one, and it
matters to me.'" —Author Unknown

John first shared this poem with me many years ago. It inspired
me then, and it still inspires me. It motivates me to consider the
everyday things that I do. The poem makes me think that...

When a task seems overwhelming, just start with the next step.

There were a million sea stars stranded on the beach, and what
did the young boy do? Instead of feeling like he was faced with an
impossible task, he just focused on the next one he could help. Starting
cancer treatment feels like an impossible task. It's so overwhelming.
There's a whole new vocabulary to learn, all sorts of tests and
procedures, and it's all so very scary. I was looking at surgeries and
treatments that would last more than a year, and as far as I was
concerned, it might as well have been forever. I didn't know what was
going to happen. I felt like everything I ever knew to be true had
disappeared overnight. So what did I do? I did what the young boy did.

I focused on taking the next step, then the next one, and the next one. And I did it, one step—one sea star—at a time.

Small gestures can make a big difference.

A sea star stranded on the beach will die. And yet how simple is it for this young boy to pick it up and toss it back into the sea? It is a small gesture for him, one he would probably be doing anyway, with rocks or pieces of driftwood. And yet that simple gesture is saving a life. Sometimes the smallest gestures are the most effective. I know from personal experience that the little gestures make a huge difference—a text message on my way to treatment, a card in the mail, a handmade greeting from young cousins, a hug, a smile—those are the things that can change the course of my day. And I realize that I can do the same for others, even when I'm feeling sick or tired or scared. Smiling at the person walking past me, saying hello to the cashier at the store, holding the door open for a mom and her baby; each gesture may be small by itself, but each one matters, each one makes a difference.

Keep doing what matters to me, regardless of what others say.

I'll bet the author of this poem wasn't the first person to ask the young boy, "Why do you waste your time this way?" There will always be people questioning what I am doing and offering advice. But once I was diagnosed with cancer, I became very good at figuring out what matters and what doesn't. Time with family and friends—matters. Time scrubbing toilets—does not matter. One more game of cribbage matters. Doing the dishes tonight—does not matter. Wrapping things up to spend time with my husband—matters. Arguing about whatever—does not matter. Doing what matters to me means listening to my inner voice, hearing what my heart is saying. It's the chance to spend my time doing the things that are meaningful to me, letting guilt and obligation become things of the past. There has always been a finite amount of time, and now I am learning to spend my time wisely—on the people and activities that matter to me.

Puzzle Piece

Week 5

This charm was chosen by me.
Why? What is happening now is one small part of
my life's picture.

I love putting a jigsaw puzzle together. There's a sense of satisfaction from taking a box of strangely cut pieces and putting them together to make a delightful picture. I feel a little like that right now. I was handed this box of odd pieces, and now I'm putting them together to create a beautiful and blessed picture.

The thing about a real jigsaw puzzle, though, is that I can choose the one I want. Do I want 100, 500, 750, or 1000 pieces? (Or maybe just a 24-piece one.) Do I want a picture that's just a collection of white flowers? Or do I want a picture with lots of colors and distinct objects? Do I want a puzzle where all the pieces are exactly the same shape? Or do I want a variety of shapes? When I choose a puzzle to put together, I can choose just what I want. I like that.

But that's not life. And it's certainly not life with cancer. I felt like I was handed a blank box filled with all these puzzle pieces. At first, all I could do was look at them and cry. How would they all go together? Where's the picture of the completed puzzle? What if some pieces were missing? But when I was done crying, it was time to take stock, to look at what was in front of me. So I picked up the pieces and started to sort them—edge pieces, pieces of similar colors or types—and I realized that putting this puzzle together was just a matter of taking one piece at a time, looking at it, appreciating it, and considering where it might fit into my life's puzzle.

"There are no extra pieces in the universe. Everyone is here because he or she has a place to fill, and every piece must fit itself into the big jigsaw puzzle."
—Deepak Chopra

There are no extra pieces. I like that thought. Every piece I collect along my journey through life fits into my unique picture puzzle. Some pieces are fairly plain, some have lots of detail, others are blurry, some are simple, some are complicated and jagged. But each one is uniquely mine, created for my puzzle alone. I may not really want one of my puzzle pieces, but that one piece could be the one that connects me to a new and beautiful part of my life. Without that one piece, my puzzle would be incomplete and not nearly as gorgeous and real.

I love it when I'm working on a puzzle that's mostly completed, and I pick up a piece that's very distinctive—perhaps it has one corner that's solid red. I'll look all over the puzzle trying to find where it goes, thinking it has to be obvious—how can I miss that red corner? Then I'll try it in a spot that's at least the right shape, figuring it's worth a try, and it fits. And it's completely right. I can't believe that I didn't see it right away, because it fits perfectly.

Or I'm trying to put the sky together. At some point I just start trying pieces, whether I think they go or not. I'm always surprised when they actually fit. Or, I put two pieces together, and I want them to fit, they mostly look like they'll fit, so I leave them. The only problem is—the rest of the puzzle won't work. I have to let the pieces fall into their places; I can't force them to fit. I can't force the things that happen in my life to fit what I want or what I planned or even what I hoped for. Each piece fits where it's supposed to fit.

I think of all the pieces I've collected over the years and the way they go together to make up the picture puzzle of me. Every person, every event in my life has given me a piece, and as I've traveled through the years, I've put them in place to create my unique and wonderful and crazy and unpredictable picture puzzle of my life.

Penguin
Week 6

This charm was chosen by me.
Why? Penguins are my husband's favorite animal,
so I chose this charm in honor of him.

Having cancer is many things, but probably one of the most universal and overwhelming things is that cancer is anxiety-producing. Cancer strikes such fear in our hearts. More women die every year of heart disease, but being diagnosed with high blood pressure doesn't evoke the same level of fear and apprehension that a breast cancer diagnosis does. From that first visit with my surgeon, the anxiety began to build. When she called with the results of the core biopsy, "You definitely have invasive ductal carcinoma in situ," but continued to explain that she wanted to do an incisional biopsy because she felt there was more going on, the anxiety increased. The feeling of being thrust into unfamiliar territory was terrifying. The anti-anxiety medicine helped, a little, but it didn't really address the core issues. The anxiety was there, yes, but there was also anger (Why is this happening to me?), fear (Am I going to die?), worry (How can I help my family deal with this?), and tears, lots and lots of tears. And then, one Sunday, my husband went to church.

The pastor that day preached about fear and anxiety, love and light. He explained that fear and anxiety are the opposite of faith, and that love and light and hope are faith embodied. I am so very grateful John went to church that particular Sunday. Those words touched his soul. And because they became a part of him, he was able to share them with me. He was able to support me and love me and lift me up. When my anxiety would start to take over, he would gently bring me back to faith and hope, light and love. It wasn't easy. There were many nights when the anxiety threatened to take over, to cover me in darkness, and the only thing I could do was cling to his love and his light and to let his faith carry me for a while.

There may be other times in my life when fear and anxiety will seem like my only option, but I know now that they are not. No matter what is happening, regardless of how dark things seem from where I am, I can always choose the light of love and faith.

I felt the darkness all around me.

I needed to run, stomp my feet, scream.

I wanted to escape, to be anywhere but here.

And then I felt his strong arms around me, quieting my fears.

Gently showing me another way,

Leading me to the light of love and faith.

—Gayle Bittinger

Fortune Cookie
Week 7

This charm was chosen by my husband, John, and me.
Why? John and I go to our favorite Chinese restaurant after every chemo treatment, where I eat my fill of Chicken Chow Mein and Lemon Chicken.

My family and I love traditions. Not for the "that's the way we've always done it" part, but for the looking forward to, anticipation part. Easter is this weekend, and I'm looking forward to Easter baskets, church, Easter dinner, and, of course, Egg Ball. (What's Egg Ball, you ask? Think baseball with hard-cooked Easter eggs in place of the ball!) This year, Easter also means time with our daughter, Katie, and her friend Cheryl, which means cooking and baking together, playing games, watching movies, and just hanging out.

When I hear the word "tradition," I think of Tevia from the musical *Fiddler on the Roof* extolling the virtues of "Tradition!" He wants things to stay the same because that's the way they've always been. But things do not stay the same, no matter how much I'd like them to. Life happens and brings with it changes that make me happy and changes that scare the living daylights out of me. Allowing my traditions to change as my life changes gives me comfort and support for whatever life brings.

I think of traditions as living, growing things. I can adapt them to my life right now. But even though the actual traditions can change, the comfort they provide is constant. One of my favorite traditions right now is the snuggle I get from John every night before we fall asleep. Sometimes we talk, often we just hold each other quietly. He'll rub my bald head or hold me extra close if I've got the shivers. And even though I'm hoping that I won't always have a bald head to rub, I know that John will always be there to hold me.

My son, Alex, and I started a fun, after-school tradition of watching episodes of the TV show *Numbers*. I don't have the energy to go outside and toss the football around or shoot some hoops, so we found a new way to connect and spend time together. I've also worked out some long-distance traditions with my daughter, Katie, who's away at college—a letter or package in the mail each week, coffee and shopping when she's home, texting in-between. I email family and friends a "Kick Some Cancer Butt (KSCB) Gazette" after every treatment to let them know how I'm doing. I meet my friend Robbie every other week for coffee and catching up.

Traditions ground us. They comfort us and connect us with the people who are important to us. Traditions remind us of where we came from and who we are. I think they are even more important when going through a life-altering diagnosis like cancer. There is comfort in knowing that no matter what else happens today, I'll have that snuggle with John, that Alex and I will watch an episode of *Numbers*, that Katie is a mere text message away. And I know that as I work through my treatments and start the healing process, our lives will change again, and our traditions will be there, waiting to adapt; waiting to find new ways to ground us, comfort us, and connect us.

Tree

This charm was chosen by my family and me.
Why? It reminds us of family, roots, growing,
life, branches, fruit, and shade.

I love trees of all kinds—evergreen trees, deciduous trees, fruit trees. The cedars on the California coast last summer were amazing—giant, majestic, gorgeous. I love the bright green buds on the deciduous trees in the spring. I spent many falls "helping" my great-grandfather with his apple harvest. To me, a tree represents sturdiness, growth, family, and belief in a God who can turn a tiny acorn into a giant oak.

When my surgeon called last October to tell me I had breast cancer, I was devastated. I felt like the deciduous trees outside my window, their leaves changing colors and then falling to the ground. I felt like everything I knew to be real and true was falling away. I felt bare and exposed and vulnerable. And I didn't like it.

Eventually, though, I realized that by shedding the old, I was able to conserve my energy, to allow myself time to process what was happening to me. When I was first diagnosed with cancer, I wanted to scream, run, keep busy, and give denial a try. But when I was forced to slow down, when I felt my leaves shedding, when I felt bare and vulnerable, the pretenses fell away and I started looking for what is real, what is me. And I discovered that I could be stronger than I ever thought I could be.

The aggressive chemotherapy and bilateral mastectomy were the first steps to shedding my cancer. Now I've started a second round of chemotherapy and a year of biotherapy infusions. I consider this the pruning phase, trimming the extra branches and training the ones that are left to grow in the best possible way. The radiation treatments this summer will be like the thinning they do with fruit trees so that the fruit that's left will be the best possible.

And next fall, as I'm working my way through the final months of biotherapy infusions, the leaves will fall again. This time, as they fall, they'll take away the last parts of the "old" me, the "I should" me, the unauthentic me. And only the real me will remain.

Growing is changing.
It is losing your leaves of hurt and pain.
It is being vulnerable as you heal,
Waiting for new growth, new hope, new life.

Growing is changing.
It is pruning your branches of doubt and fear.
It is thinning out the unauthentic,
Waiting for buds of joy and celebration to appear.

—Gayle Bittinger

Gift

This charm was chosen by me.
Why? Every day is a gift.

When I unwrapped the "gift" of my breast cancer diagnosis, I expected to find fear, anxiety, uncertainty, worry, and lots of doctor appointments. And I did find those. But have you ever gotten a gift wrapped inside a gift wrapped inside a gift? That's what having cancer is like. I unwrapped the first gift, and it was filled will all those things I'd expected—fear of the unknown, anxiety over what will happen, worries about test results, and lots and lots of appointments. But, I also discovered another gift to unwrap.

When I unwrapped that second gift, I found the challenge of telling my family and friends about my diagnosis. This was a gift of tears and hugs, as the people who loved me were drawn into my story. It has also been a gift of prayers and support because reaching out to others has given me the strength to face whatever comes next. It has been a gift overflowing with love and caring, kindness and generosity, warm meals delivered to our home, cards in the mail. It continues to be the gift that keeps me going, the one that helps me get from one treatment to the next. This gift reminds me that I am loved. It is the gift that encourages me and lifts my spirit.

The final gift I unwrapped was the one I am still giving to myself. This gift is filled with the treasures I am collecting on this journey: treasures I may have never discovered if I hadn't been diagnosed with cancer. That is a humbling thought. I can't say I was happy to be handed the "gift" of a cancer diagnosis, but I can honestly say it has been a blessing in my life. Being diagnosed and treated for cancer has helped me discover things about myself I'm not sure I would have ever figured out. It has helped me grow and change. It has helped me focus my energies and discern what is truly important to me.

There were times when I looked at this gift

And wondered if I could get a full refund

If I had only kept my receipt.

But as it turns out,

There was no receipt, no return, no refund.

Instead I found this gift was

All I truly needed—

Love and friendship,

Grace and forgiveness,

Patience and empathy,

Gratitude and appreciation,

Faith and hope,

And I found myself with a gift I will keep forever.

—Gayle Bittinger

Flower

This charm was chosen by me.
Why? A flower represents spring, growth,
and beauty.

"A real friend is one who overlooks the broken-down
gate and admires the flowers in your garden."
—Author Unknown

This dear friend doesn't try to fix my gate or offer to help me fix it or gingerly step through it. My real friend overlooks—probably doesn't even see—the broken gate, and is captivated by what is truly valuable, beautiful, treasured. How many times do we try to "fix" a friend, to patch up that broken-down gate? Or maybe to judge just a little bit, to compare gates, so to speak. Being a true friend is so much more than accepting someone as he or she is. It's about finding, seeing, and appreciating the special qualities unique in each of us. Getting caught up in what's wrong, what needs to be fixed, is easy. What's difficult is seeing the beauty beyond the brokenness, the flowers beyond the gate.

When I think of a garden with a broken-down gate, I see a white picket fence, a bit shabby, with a gate opened and hanging from one hinge. There's a path that leads into a lush, somewhat overgrown garden bursting with blooms of all colors, shapes, and sizes. There's a bench with a bird bath and feeder close by. I feel like the garden is inviting me in. I feel like I could sit and enjoy the garden there, or I could cut some flowers and take their joy and sunshine with me.

Cancer is like the broken-down gate. It's right there, front and center in my life. I can't get away from it. The treatments and side effects remind me daily, sometimes hourly, that I have cancer. Some days it feels like everything I do is about my cancer—treatments and side effects, appointments and phone calls, and lots and lots of naps—it's hard see anything but the cancer.

This broken-down gate, my cancer, is also the first thing many others see. There are times when I long for someone to see beyond the gate, to see the colors and blooms in the garden of my life. I am a woman who is being treated for breast cancer. I am a woman who is a wife, a mother, a daughter, a sister, an aunt, a friend. I am a woman who loves to spend time with family and friends, to write and create, bake and sew. I am more than my breast cancer. I am separate from my cancer. I want people to look beyond my cancer—beyond my broken-down gate—to see the real me, to see the beauty and color and life I have inside of me.

It's important for me to remember who I am beyond my cancer, to keep the essential me alive. Cancer has changed me, there's no doubt about that. My garden will never be the same. It will be better. I will find new and wonderful flowers to plant in my garden. I will find a pair of comfortable chairs to put in the middle of my garden. I may even find a new appreciation and love for that broken-down gate, but it will always be my garden—before, during, and after cancer.

Sometimes it is so hard
To remember who I am.
I am not my cancer.

I am not
My chemotherapy,
My surgery,
My infusions,
My radiation.

I am a woman who is
Being treated for breast cancer.

I am a woman who is
A wife, a mother, a daughter,
A sister, an aunt, a friend.

I am a woman who is
Happy and sad,
Strong and weak,
Angry and content,
Anxious and calm.

I am me—
Just me, only me, always me.

—Gayle Bittinger

Hummingbird
Week 11

This charm was chosen by my husband, John. Why? "It reminds me of the hummingbird on the card I gave you."

The Mother's Day card my husband chose for me this year reminded me of several things I'd like to make time for every day.

Discovering Beauty

Beauty isn't the packaged product Madison Avenue would like us to believe it is. Beauty isn't found in a bottle, a potion, or a store. It isn't something to put on. Beauty is everywhere. It is the essence, the heart, the core of something or someone. It is the intricacy of a snowflake, the grandeur of a mountain range, the power of the ocean, the grace of a dancer, the love of a spouse, the joy of a child, the steadfastness of a friend. All I need to do to discover the beauty that surrounds me is to open my heart and my eyes.

Appreciating Connections

The connections we make with others—that's what life is about. When I think of the connections that led me to this moment in time, many stand out; others are smaller, but still essential; and some, I know, are hidden or forgotten. But every connection has value. Every connection has given my life meaning, creating the framework for love and hope and faith.

Remembering to Laugh

I love to laugh. I love to share a giggle, a chuckle, a belly laugh, or a laugh so hard I can barely catch my breath. Sometimes my daughter and I will laugh until we cry. Sharing a laugh breaks down walls, creates connections, celebrates beauty, and highlights the richness of my life. My family makes me laugh. That was one of the first things I noticed about John and one of the many reasons I fell in love with him. He makes me laugh every day. And one of the great joys of life is the first time you hear your child let loose with a giant belly laugh. It is such a joyful sound. Laughter is a way to rejoice and celebrate life.

Living Each Day

I want to be present every day, basking in moments of beauty, appreciating my connections with others, and remembering to laugh with love, joy, and celebration.

Each day I have a choice to
Delight in the abundance of my life—

To know the joy of sitting at the table with my family,
Sharing a meal we've prepared together.

To feel the blessing of waking up beside my beloved every morning.
To experience the comfort of familiar routines.

To appreciate the satisfaction of being a part of something bigger than myself.
To celebrate God's love in all of creation.

—Gayle Bittinger

Pumpkin Carriage
Week 12

This charm was chosen by me.
Why? I am learning to trust my journey.

Of all the encouraging and inspiring quotes I've read and received the past eight months, these three words have been the most meaningful and powerful to me: Trust Your Journey.

Trust

I am learning to trust myself and to trust that the steps I am taking will lead me to healing and wholeness. So I trust that what I'm experiencing is real for me, and I choose my journey based on those experiences. I trust that each step I take is the one I am meant to take. I trust that each day I am where I am meant to be, doing what I need to do.

Your

This is my journey, and I am the one in charge of the itinerary. Do I need something along the way? I can let others know. Do I have a question? I can ask. Do I need some time to consider my next step or to just take a breath? I can do that. And I don't have to follow in anyone else's footsteps. It is my journey. I can choose if my next step is big or small, if I want to turn right or left, if I'm going to ask for directions or explore on my own. It is my journey to take, but I am, oh, so thankful for family, friends, and providers who are walking with me, letting me lead the way, helping me over the obstacles, and encouraging me to keep taking that next step.

Journey

I had no idea what kind of journey I was embarking on when I made that first appointment with my family practitioner because I just wasn't feeling right. It's probably just as well. Then there was that first meeting with my surgeon. She knew what journey I was about to take, or was at least pretty certain. And although the journey wasn't up to me, I am choosing how I travel. I am focusing on not only healing my body, but also my spirit. I am becoming me. I am unpacking the guilt and leaving it behind. I am taking time for what's important. I'm enjoying the trip and all of the blessings I've discovered along the way.

Trust your journey.

It may not be the journey of your choice,

But it can be a journey that takes you from

Sickness to health,

Despair to hope,

Tears to laughter,

Frenzy to peace,

Rushing to relaxing,

Doing to being.

—Gayle Bittinger

Crown

This charm was chosen by Marlene, my nurse practitioner at Columbia Basin Hematology and Oncology. Why? "You've tolerated everything we've given you so well, you deserve a crown."

"Princesses wear crowns to remind them that they are smart and beautiful, because some days it's easy to forget." —Author Unknown

I feel like I need a crown these days. It's easy to forget that I'm smart when the chemo brain kicks in and I spend twenty minutes looking for the gloves I just took off, or I can't remember the title of a favorite book. It's also pretty easy to feel less than beautiful, when my arm feels swollen and heavy from lymphedema, my hands and feet are tingling, and I find myself in a body that feels like it's missing a few things (like breasts and hair).

Cancer is the word that knocked the crown right off my head and sent it rolling down the castle stairs. A cancer diagnosis is scary and not quite the fairy tale I imagined for myself. But after the initial shock passed, I picked up my crown, put it on, and got to work. I found incredibly kind and skilled doctors and nurses to work with, I reached out to family and friends, and I started writing a new fairy tale for myself.

And all of a sudden, I realized that I had an opportunity. I'd been given a chance to look at my life, to choose what I wanted to include in my story and what I wanted to leave out. I had the opportunity to start living in the moment, to make joy, love, and contentment my everyday reality, and to leave anger, frustration, and impatience behind. It was a chance for me to let go of worrying about what others were thinking and doing the things that were meaningful to me.

It's amazing how a crown can help me feel more like myself. Not that I haven't wallowed here and there when I felt overwhelmed or scared or afraid of losing something. But it doesn't really suit me to wallow or feel down, so I put on my crown. It's like my morning routine. Every morning, regardless of how I feel, I get up, get dressed, put on some make-up, and don my imaginary crown. It's a little thing, but I feel so much better. Life is so much more livable when I feel like being up and about. Actually, it's more livable when I AM up and about—whether I feel like it or not.

As a crown-wearing princess, I must remember to move at a slow and regal pace, taking one chapter at a time, even though there are days when I would just like to skip to the happily ever after. Instead, I picture myself at the end of this fairy tale, feeling more like myself than I have in a long time—with my crown firmly in place. I am the princess who tells the tale of how my prince and I are slaying the dragon with the help of an entire kingdom. I am the princess who puts on her crown and chooses to live with joy, love, and contentment every day. I am the princess who is blessed with the support of family, friends, and caregivers. I am the princess who is writing her own Happily Ever After.

The Letter B

This charm was chosen by me.
Why? Life is all about how you handle Plan B.

Wouldn't it be nice if you could just follow Plan A your whole life, happy and content with the way things are? Nice, but not very realistic. Plan A is usually the comfortable and familiar plan, the one that rarely lasts very long. Plan B is what makes life... Interesting! Exciting! Scary! Surprising! Terrifying! Exhilarating! Amazing! Worthwhile!

Plan B makes you stop and think. Plan B includes a touch of the unknown with a bit of the scary. What do you do when you have to go to Plan B? Do you embrace the scary parts and open yourself up to grace and miracles? Do you let yourself live in a state of peaceful unpredictability? Do you worry about every possibility? Or do you let go and just be? How do you find balance when your whole world has been knocked out of kilter?

When all of your plans have gone cattywompus, you finally have the opportunity to realize that you are not in control. When all you are left with is Plan B, you can move from going through the motions to living each day. From the usual routine to special occasion. From mismatched plates to Grandma's china. From vanilla to "death by chocolate." From reruns to series' premieres. From meat and potatoes to Rachel Ray's Grilled Flank Steak and Asparagus on Puff Pastry Squares. From store-bought produce to home-grown bites of deliciousness. From the rush of the everyday to the quiet of being at peace. From instant coffee to espresso. From a game of solitaire to seven rousing rounds of Progressive Rummy with family and friends.

From a walk around the block to a hike through the woods to a hidden lake.

How do you feel when all of your plans go sideways? Perhaps just a little scared, mixed in with some anticipation, a bit of worry that you won't know what to do, dusted with the excitement of something new. Mostly, though, Plan B calls us to action. Plan B gives us an opportunity to start anew. Plan B reminds us that life is to be lived outside the lines. Plan B is where miracles and blessings flow.

Plan B is Beautiful, Big, Boisterous,

Bliss, Brassy, Bubbly,

Brash, Bonkers, Bright,

Bittersweet, Bountiful, Bewildering,

Baffling, Bouncy, Brainy,

Brave, Breezy, Beastly,

Beguiling, Boundless, Bold,

Brilliant, Brazen, and Blessed.

—Gayle Bittinger

Dragonfly
Week 15

This charm was chosen by my friend Heather.
Why? "My friend Dina had breast cancer, and
dragonflies were her inspiration."

North American Indians consider the dragonfly to be the "essence of the winds of change." I can understand why someone who has been diagnosed with cancer would choose a dragonfly as inspiration. Having cancer is nothing but change—a change in how I see myself, a change in how I view my mortality, a change in my view of what's important and what's not, a change in what I can do, a change in how I spend my time, a change in how I feel physically, a change in how independent I am. Cancer is change.

Change is scary.

I liked the way things were going before I was diagnosed with cancer. I mostly knew what to expect. I could do the things I wanted to do. Life with cancer is scary.

Change is hard.

I enjoyed knowing what to expect, having an idea of how my days would go. Now there are so many appointments, infusions, surgeries, radiation treatments, lymphatic therapy sessions, side effects. It seems like my days are filled with cancer treatments. Life with cancer is hard.

Change is anxiety-producing.

What will the treatments be like? How will I deal with the side effects? Will I survive? Will my family and friends be ok? Life with cancer is filled with anxiety.

And...Change is opportunity.

It's a chance to see life with new eyes. Having cancer brings my life into focus. I don't have time for pretense; I value what's real and meaningful. Life with cancer is opportunity.

Change is adventure.

If adventure means travelling down a path I never thought I'd take, then having cancer is definitely an adventure. I have met so many amazing, caring people on this adventure: people I would have never had the privilege of knowing without a cancer diagnosis. Life with cancer is an adventure.

Change is life.

There will always be change. What I do with that change is what matters. Having cancer changed my life and the lives of the people who love and care for me. When I embrace that change, when I allow it to sweep through my life, I understand that what I do with that change is entirely up to me. Life with cancer is... life.

After the winds of change blow through

You are left with a sense of being swept clean.

You find that the unnecessary and the extraneous

Have disappeared in the zephyr.

And all that remains is what is real,

What is meaningful,

What is you.

—Gayle Bittinger

Guardian Angel
Week 16

This charm was chosen by Hanane, one of my infusion nurses at Columbia Basin Hematology and Oncology.
Why? "So you will always have an angel watching over you."

An angel to watch over me...To be honest, I've had some trouble with this. What does it mean to have an angel watching over me? If the cancer returns, does that mean I didn't believe enough? Or deserve enough? I guess it comes back to what I struggled with in the beginning, that human and eternal question, "Why me?" I wondered if it was all "part of God's plan for me," and then I thought, "Well, if that's true, then God's plan stinks!"

I prefer looking at my cancer from the perspective of Rabbi Harold S. Kushner in his book *When Bad Things Happen to Good People.* "The God I believe in does not send us the problem; He gives us the strength to cope with the problem." This is an imperfect world. I didn't get cancer because I wasn't good enough or because I'm strong enough to handle it or because God wanted me to have it for some reason known only to Him. But I also know that God has been with me from that first scary phone call. He's been there through appointments, chemotherapy, surgery, and more chemotherapy. I can reach out to God when I need encouragement or strength or patience. I feel God's presence in every moment, holding me up, walking beside me. The author of the poem, "Footprints" knew that. God can't keep the tough times from happening, but, if I ask, God will walk every difficult step with me, even carry me, if necessary.

Everything that has happened because of my cancer—feeling closer to my husband than ever, spending time with my family, connecting with friends, eating delicious meals made just for us, receiving cards and greetings from the people in my life, being treated by skilled and compassionate providers—that's where I see God's hand, working through my life and the lives of the people who care for me.

If I understand that a guardian angel is a person who looks after or cares about someone else, then this angel charm on my necklace is really a symbol of the dozens of guardian angels I already have watching over me. And, I must admit, I need reminders that God is close, that I am loved, that my life has meaning. As I work through my treatments, however, the thought of the cancer returning is a little daunting, and more than a little scary. But I am choosing to keep a positive attitude. I am choosing to allow my angels to do their jobs— loving and caring for me, showing me how to enjoy each day, and reminding me to live, not in fear, but in joy.

Treble Clef
Week 17

This charm was chosen by my son, Alex.
Why? "For no particular reason, because
sometimes we just need to do things for no
particular reason."

To me, the treble clef represents music, and when I think of music, I certainly think of my children, Alex and Katie. Music has always inspired them. Katie attended a music camp where this was the theme:

Why talk when you can sing?
Why walk when you can dance?

That's my family. Why do something in a plain and ordinary way, when it can be done with joy and verve and life? What a great way to approach life. Sometimes there isn't a choice about what happens or what must be done, but there is always a choice about how it's approached or handled. Everyday things become special if I shift the way I look at them just a little bit...

Do I heat up baked beans or Serve Cowboy Caviar?

Do I hop in the tub or Soak in the Bath?

Do I throw dinner together or Feed My Family?

Do I cross things off my to-do list or Enjoy My Accomplishments?

Do I get soaked in the drizzle or Dance in the Rain?

It comes back to the question, "Is your glass half empty or half full?" I can choose to approach each day as if my glass is half empty—

just another day to get through with a myriad of shoulds and to dos. Or, I can choose a half-full attitude and look at each day as a gift, a present to unwrap with anticipation and excitement.

Why talk when you can SING?
Why walk when you can DANCE?

Lately, there's been a little more talking and walking in my life than I'd like. The treatments mean my constant companions are fatigue, neuropathy, GI distress, hot flashes, and chemo brain. It's hard to remember to sing and dance when I'm wearing a tank top for the hot flashes and wool socks and gloves for the neuropathy, when nothing sounds good to eat, when I can't for the life of me remember where I set down my cup of tea, and all I want to do is take a nap! These are the times when it's even more essential for me to remember that the singing and the dancing are what make everything else worthwhile.

So, it's time for me to approach each day with a song in my heart and a spring in my step. There are no more plain and ordinary days for me. Each day is an opportunity to take care of myself and my family. Each day I have the ability to choose joy and happiness. Each day is a chance to be with people who lift my spirit. Each day gives me possibilities to ask for what I need and to ask how I can help nurture and nourish others. Each day is a gift I can open with singing and dancing.

Butterfly
Week 18

This charm was chosen by me.
Why? I feel like a butterfly, emerging from
its cocoon.

"It takes courage to grow up and become who you
really are." —e.e. cummings

If I want to grow up and become who I really am, I will need
not only courage, but also determination, vision, resolution, and pluck.
I am developing these qualities as I travel on my journey from cancer
diagnosis through treatment into healing and wholeness.

It takes **COURAGE** to grow up and become who I really am,
to do the things that are essential for me. It is particularly poignant
today because I have chosen to have my radiation treatments in
Spokane, a city more than two hours away from home. Sometimes
what I need or what is best for me isn't necessarily what's best or
easiest or convenient for everyone else in my family. And even if my
family doesn't mind, even if my family agrees that radiation treatment
in Spokane is best and is willing to work around my new summer
schedule, it's still hard for me to put myself and my needs first. Going
to a new city without the comforts of home is a little scary for me. But
when I act with courage, I am able to take a risk, follow my instincts,
and do something different. With courage, I can grow up to become
who I really am.

It takes **DETERMINATION** to grow up and be true to myself
and my needs. When I have determination, I have a firmness of
purpose. And I do have a new firmness of purpose—healing and
wholeness. Everything I do to care for myself—eating healthfully,

exercising and being active, nourishing my mental health—brings healing into my life. When I act with determination, I am able to focus on what's important without distractions. With determination, I can grow up to become who I really am.

It takes **VISION** and wisdom to imagine the person I can be, the person I want to be. What is my vision for myself? That's probably the toughest question of all. I'm a writer. I'm a wife and a mother, a daughter and a sister. I love to bake, and I'm learning to love to cook. I do love the outdoors, especially early morning just after the sun rises and at night when the stars are out. I love to travel and explore. I'm a reader. I'm a friend. I am a person who lives life to the fullest. And with vision, I can find a way to honor my strengths and interests as I grow up to become who I really am.

It takes **RESOLUTION** to become who I am. It means hanging in there, getting up when I fall or stumble. It means that the end— becoming who I really am—is worth the means. It means taking the time to rethink my priorities, to examine my short-term and long-term goals. Resolution means getting up each day and starting where I am. It means that even if it feels like three steps forward and two steps back, I am making progress. With resolution, I understand that each baby step I take is important and valuable as I grow up and become who I really am.

It takes **PLUCK** and a desire to grow into the person I am meant to be... the person I want to be... the person I long to be. I am beginning this journey to become who I am meant to be with joy, with the certainty that I am doing what I am meant to be doing, and with anticipation for what each moment will bring as I grow up and become who I really am.

Locket

This charm was chosen by me.
Why? I put photos of my family in the locket
because my family means the world to me.

I know that my breast cancer is hard on my family. It's tough to know that someone you love is sick with what is still considered to be a pretty scary disease. When I was first diagnosed, my husband, John, said that one of his first thoughts was that he wished it were he so I wouldn't have to go through all the treatments and side effects and surgeries. But then he said he realized that if he were the one with cancer, I'd be the one by his side worrying and feeling helpless—and he wouldn't wish that on me or anyone. Quite an insight into the difficulty of being a bystander in all of this, and yet he has been there through everything—appointments, treatments, surgery, tears, frustrations, mood swings, despair, joy, setbacks, success. I truly can't imagine doing this without him.

Family is important any time, but they are essential when dealing with a life-altering illness. However, as I am learning, I must find other baskets for my "eggs." I can't expect my family to fulfill all of my emotional needs. That's true during normal, everyday life; it's even truer now. So, besides my delightfully loving and supportive family, I am relying on my friends. I've never been one to have lots of easy friendships. I have a few really good friends and a variety of casual acquaintances that pop in and out of my life. I've always wondered why I couldn't seem to manage the large group of friends—wondering what was wrong with me, to be honest—and then my dear friend Cyndi sent me a poem about girlfriends that explained how some friends enter your life for a season, others for life. That is a much healthier way for me to look at what sometimes seems like a revolving door for acquaintances—to see them not as failures, but as "seasons."

It's what Dorothy Gilman writes in her mystery novel *The Clairvoyant Countess*, "If you could only turn the kaleidoscope a fraction of an inch the view would dazzle you!" When a friendship's season comes to an end, I can be thankful for the time together and allow it to be a time remembered fondly, instead of kicking myself for not being a better friend or wondering what happened or thinking there's something wrong with me. In this particular case, I need to be more like a guy...

One of the guys at my house made instant mashed potatoes last week. They were really runny. It was pretty obvious that this particular guy had misread the chart on the back of the box and used the water for six servings and the potatoes for four, but he said, "I don't know what's wrong with the potatoes. I followed the directions." No guilt. No wondering what he did wrong. The problem was with the potatoes. I remember wishing I could do that. Computer file AWOL? Obviously the computer did it. Trip over a step? Give it a kick. It's not personal. That's a good reminder for me. I'm all too fast blaming myself or thinking I've done something wrong. I must remember that some things just are.

Turn the kaleidoscope
And stop blaming yourself for
Friendships that fizzle,
Recipes that flop,
Computer files that crash,
And, most importantly,
A diagnosis of breast cancer.

Some things just are and they are
NOT YOUR FAULT.
Turn the kaleidoscope...
The view just might dazzle you.

—Gayle Bittinger

Three Keys
Week 20

This charm was chosen by my friend LaLani.
Why? "So we can always remember our exciting,
if not stressful, housing arrangements for this
first week of radiation treatments."

My dear friend LaLani had the privilege of being the first chaperone for my radiation treatments at Cancer Care Northwest in Spokane (about 150 miles from my home). We had a great week, even if our housing arrangements were a little "fly by the seat of your pants." LaLani was my key to a wonderful first week. And she inspired me to think about what's key to me, what makes a difference in how I see and approach life.

One of the things I've learned since being diagnosed with cancer is that life is too short to spend time trying to change the people I love. How many times have I wished that a loved one would be more (fill-in-the-blank) or maybe a little less (fill-in-the-blank)? It's a natural thing to do, but when I start trying to change the people in my life, all I'm guaranteed to get is disappointment and tears. I can't change someone else. The only thing I can do is love the people in my life and trust that they are the people they are meant to be right now.

That's a tough one—trusting people to be who they are rather than changing them into who I want them to be. And even though it's difficult, amazing things happen when I trust people to be who they are. I see their true gifts, their unique qualities. I see them as they are, warts and all. I see where they excel and where they struggle. I see their hopes and dreams, their fears and worries. When I start looking at the people in my life with clear eyes, I find qualities I never imagined.

When I see them with my heart, I trust them to be who they are, without judgment, without wishful thinking, without agenda.

When I look at people with expectations for them to behave in certain ways, I'm in for tears—guaranteed. And what makes those tears especially heartbreaking is that if I were to look at them as they truly are, I would be surprised. In fact, I would most likely be thrilled. Sometimes I am so busy trying to get the people in my life to be who I want them to be, that I forget to see them as they truly are. And they truly are amazing.

Perhaps there's a woman who has just had an anxiety-producing visit with a new oncologist, and she wishes her husband would tell her that everything will be ok, that all of these new tests and procedures are the result of a doctor being cautious, not an unfortunate example of too little too late. Her husband is worried, scared. He's angry that he didn't think of those things months ago. He is frustrated that he wasn't able to protect her. He doesn't have any words he can say out loud right now. All he can do is hold her, wrap his arms around her, love her. But she misses it because she thinks she wants something else. In fact, she is so focused on that something else, she misses the love and concern that's right in front of her... that was right in front of me.

I've spent more time than I care to admit wishing people were behaving differently, wishing they would act the way I wanted them to act. I'm learning that the world is a much better place when I trust people to be who they are. Each person has a distinct point of view, a unique set of gifts to offer. When I take the time to see the people in my life as they truly are and to trust them to be the amazing, wonderful, and fabulous people they are, my life is richer, fuller, and much, much better.

Route 66

This charm was chosen by me.
Why? I will have traveled 2400 miles to and from
Spokane for radiation treatments this summer,
about the length of Route 66. I plan to travel those
miles on the actual Route 66 someday.

I love the idea of traveling on Route 66. Taking the slow way instead of the Interstate, stopping to enjoy all of the sights along the way, the road not taken...

"Two roads diverged in a wood, and I—I took the one
less traveled by, and that has made all the difference."
—Robert Frost

Having breast cancer has certainly put me on the road less traveled, a road that has made all the difference. How clear my life has become since coming face-to-face with my own mortality. We all know, in abstract at least, that we're going to die, but a cancer diagnosis makes that concept a lot less abstract. And that's tough to deal with, especially for family and friends, and for me as well, to be perfectly honest. It's so easy to get lost in the anxiety and worry and stress that come with having a serious disease. I prefer to keep my focus on this moment because the truth is that none of us have a guaranteed amount of time on this earth. When I am present in this moment, I see what is in front of me. I am able to enjoy my life in the here and now with what I have right now.

It is so tempting to lose myself in the busyness of life, to avoid thinking about my illness by always thinking about what's next, to keep my mind off the what ifs by racing from one activity to the next. It's like speeding along on the Interstate—I can go miles and miles and miles without having to really see anything or even stop. But when I take the road less traveled, I'm on the road I can't rush. This is the side road, the one that meanders from one town to the next. This is the road where I can get stuck behind a farm tractor going twenty miles an hour. This is the road where I slow down and truly see what's around me, where people and experiences have time to touch my heart. There's no rush on the road less traveled. I can savor each moment, each experience, each relationship.

The best thing about the road less traveled is that it is available to all of us, no matter where we are. The road less traveled is in this moment. I know I'm on it when I stop regretting what's past or worrying about what's to come. It's where I can just be. I am on the road less traveled whenever I take the time to focus on the who and the what of this moment.

I'm not saying my journey on the road less traveled is simple. In the blink of an eye I'll find myself on the Interstate of guilt and regrets, out of the moment, and away from the road less traveled. Now when I find my mind wallowing in the past or feeling anxious about the future, I know it's time to bring myself back to the present. Each day the choice is mine—do I hop on the Interstate, or do I slow down and enjoy the road less traveled? I choose to slow down, to live in the moment. I choose the road less traveled.

Star

This charm was chosen by me.
Why? I love looking at the stars on a clear night.

Stars for Friendship

I certainly don't get to see my long-distance friends as much as I'd like, but I know they are thinking of me, praying for me, keeping me in their hearts. It's comforting to know that. Having cancer can be lonely. There is lots of support at the beginning, but not everyone realizes what a long road it is. I so appreciate all of my friends, but I am especially thankful for the ones who are still here, hanging out with me and supporting me. And I must remember that my friends are always there, even if I can't see them. All I have to do is reach out.

Stars for Commitment

The stars represent constancy. Sailors navigate by them. Astronomers study them and learn about the universe. The stars shine even when they can't be seen. It's like being in a relationship. It's the constancy. It's the showing up every day. It's the commitment to shine to the best of my ability that really matters, that makes the difference.

Stars for Togetherness

Even though the stars I see each night are from hundreds of different galaxies, when I look at them, I put them together, to create familiar shapes and symbols. My perspective helps me see a particular group of stars as a whole picture. It's human nature to want to put things together, to group them. One star is pretty, but a group of stars together can make a spectacular picture.

Stars for Light

There is something magical about starlight, especially where there's very little light pollution. There are probably lots of magical experiences I miss out on because of the "pollution" in my life. I'm too frazzled, too busy, too tired, too preoccupied, too overbooked. I always want to have time to soak up the starlight and whatever magical experiences come my way.

Stars for Guidance

Jiminy Cricket said, "Always let your conscience be your guide." But what if we let starlight be our guide? What if all of us let beauty and wonder and constancy and togetherness and friendship lead the way? What an amazing world this would be.

Stars for Comfort

There is comfort in the familiar, knowing what to expect. The stars and their constellations can be seen from almost anywhere. They are continually moving, but in a way that's predictable and knowable. It's comforting to know that I can share the same sky with someone who's far away.

"I see the stars and the stars see me.
The stars see the one that I long to see.
God bless the stars and God bless me,
And God bless the one that I long to see."
—Adapted Traditional

Teapot
Week 23

This charm was chosen by my friend Robbie. Why? "As a symbol of our Hanford Friday coffee/tea dates."

"Life may not be the party we hoped for, but while we're here we should dance." —Author Unknown

For many people, life probably isn't the party they hoped for. Maybe they wanted to make more money, have a different job, live in a bigger house, get that promotion, take more vacations, look a different way, or never been diagnosed with cancer...

After I was diagnosed with breast cancer, when it became apparent that my life was not going to be the party I had hoped for, I thought that if I rushed around like Super Woman, trying to make my life look like a party I might want to attend, I'd feel like dancing. I didn't. Then I hoped that if I kept myself busy, kept moving from one task to the next, I could avoid thinking about the party at all. I thought about it. Finally, I decided to just stop for a moment and take notice of the party that was already happening. I decided to slow down and appreciate what was in front of me at that moment. And that was when I realized I could dance to the music that was already playing, that every moment of my life is an opportunity to dance.

It's hard to feel like dancing when the sink backs up and the kids are late for school and the bills need to be paid and there's no milk in the house and... I will always have things that don't go the way I'd like them to, but how many times a day do I stop to celebrate, to truly appreciate the many blessings I experience every day? Life is a celebration, and I can celebrate all of it, the good times and the bad times, the "I-hope-I-don't-have-to-do-that-again" times and the "More!" times. Each moment is an opportunity for me to celebrate.

It's amazing how often my thoughts and inspirations come back to this one simple idea—be present. Be here. Celebrate what is today. Dance, rejoice, revel in the joy of the moment. Now is the time to stop doing things out of guilt or resentment. Now is the time to start living my life. Now is the time to start making my own choices and being present with love and celebration and joy.

Life may not be the party I hoped for. That is certainly true. I can't imagine a cancer diagnosis ever being the party anyone hoped for. But can I really dance when everything I thought about the way my life would be falls apart? Absolutely, positively, yes! In fact, I believe dancing is the best way to "Embrace Plan B."

Most likely, life won't be everything you've hoped for, wanted, dreamed of, planned, charted, expected, wished for, or anticipated. And that's okay. Of course, sometimes that means a trip down a scary and uncertain road; or a big, heartfelt wish that things could have gone differently, but no matter how you got to "Life may not be the party you hoped for," the only thing left to do is relax, be present, and dance!

Koi Fish
Week 24

This charm was chosen by my friend Laurie K. Why? "There are two of them—for the two of us in Spokane, for the two Koi fish in the Japanese Garden at Manito Park, and because the fish was the first symbol of Christianity."

Peace and Tranquility

One of the first places I took Laurie to was the Japanese Garden at Spokane's Manito Park. The garden is amazing. Visitors are immersed in trees and flowers, shade and sun, ponds and walking paths, calm and quiet. It's the perfect place to visit between appointments at the cancer center. I feel a sense of peace and tranquility when I'm there. The garden has inspired me to think of ways to create spaces of peace and tranquility no matter where I am. Meditating is one way to do this. By centering myself and breathing deeply, I can let go of worries to find peace and tranquility. And it's something I can do, no matter where I am—in a crowded waiting room, in my chair in the infusion suite, or waiting in the examination room for my latest doctor's appointment.

Walking a labyrinth is another way for me to let go of my worries and to allow God's peace to flow through me. It is a way for me to connect with the holy. Walking a labyrinth is a way to literally move into peace and tranquility. It is strolling along a path with twists and turns that eventually lead me to the center. It is symbolic of the journeys we take. Have you ever started walking one way and ended up going another? That's how it feels to walk a labyrinth. I think I am almost finished, and then the path turns me away. But if I keep walking, all of a sudden, I arrive at the center, wondering how I got there. It certainly is a metaphor for life, with or without cancer. I might be able to see a little ways ahead, but I don't know for sure what's around the next corner. That uncertainty can be a blessing because it forces me to live in the moment, to appreciate what's in front of me. Yes, I can see that my path turns, but I can't change that. All I can do is enjoy where I am right now.

Love and Friendship

This Bible verse is one of Laurie K.'s favorites. "Now all glory to God, who is able, through his mighty power at work within us, to accomplish infinitely more than we might ask or think." —Eph. 3:20

There are so many people praying for my family and me. I am grateful for all of them. And I know that there are as many different prayers for me as there are people praying. It's like being wrapped in a blanket of love and hope and grace. When I pray, I find myself asking for healing and wholeness. And I see God working through me and the people in my life, providing infinitely more than any of us might ask or think.

Strength and Perseverance

With strength, I am able to withstand whatever comes my way. With perseverance, I am committed to my purpose. I have found, this past year, that I am so much stronger than I ever imagined and that my perseverance comes from greeting each new day with an open and loving heart.

With strength and perseverance I will
Seek health and healing,
Be thankful for my many blessings,
Find peace and love in every moment,
And trust in a God who is infinitely more.

—Gayle Bittinger

Elephant
Week 25

This charm was chosen by me, with the help of my husband, John. Why? It's said that elephants never forget.

I want to always remember the affirmations I've been listening to this summer. Belleruth Naparstek, co-founder of Health Journeys, has created many CDs of guided imagery and affirmations. The one I'm listening to now is filled with affirmations about healing and wholeness that have changed how I approach life.

I am letting go of expectations.

This is life changing. Letting go of expectations for myself and the people in my life to act in a certain manner or to have things go a particular way means I can relax. I can enjoy. I can be present. It allows me to make things the best they can be at that moment without worrying about meeting inflexible (and usually impossible) expectations. I can feel joy and satisfaction in doing the best job I can do right here, right now.

I am taking time to care for myself.

Taking time to care for myself used to be so very difficult for me. I had to let go of the expectation that everyone else's needs came ahead of mine. Once I did that, I was able to relax and put myself first some of the time. And I do believe that when I take the time to care for myself—preparing healthy food; walking; strengthening my body through stretches and exercises; journaling and meditating and praying—all of these activities are telling my body that I want to be healthy and well.

I am acting out of love, not guilt.

It was so nice to celebrate Christmas without guilt this past year. I was able to let go of the expectation that all gifts must be exactly fair and equitable. I was able to let go and enjoy creating gifts for family and friends out of my love for them. I allowed myself to embrace the joy of the season. Now, I can't imagine celebrating Christmas any other way. When I do things out of love and celebration, they are easy to do.

I am inviting others to help me.

I must remember that I am not alone. There are many people—friends, family, providers—who are willing to help me. Reaching out to them reminds me that this is a journey I do not have to walk alone. It does not mean that I am not strong enough or smart enough or able enough to do what needs to be done. It means that I know there is strength in numbers.

I am focusing on this moment.

Near the end of the track, Belleruth recites this affirmation, "More and more I can understand that I can heal myself and live, or I can heal myself and die. My physical condition is not an indication of my wholeness." At first, whenever I heard that, I would imagine putting my hands over my ears chanting, "I'm not listening, I'm not listening." I was afraid if I actually "heard" the words, I would be overwhelmed with sadness. Eventually, though, I understood that what she was saying was true. The outcome is out of my control. All I can do is focus on my healing and wholeness in this moment.

When my mind is wrapped up in worries of mortality,
I can't see the beauty of this day.

When I fret about how little time I might have,
I can't hear the laughter of my children.

When fears of dying fill my thoughts,
I can't feel the love that is all around me.

But when I let go of my worries,
My anxieties, my fears,

When I embrace healing and wholeness,
Without regard to my physical condition,

I experience the beauty and laughter and love in my life.
I experience the miracle of being alive.

—Gayle Bittinger

Turtle

This charm was chosen by Tess, my counselor at Cancer Care Northwest. Why? "Let the beauty of being forced to slow down be a blessing."

Tess explains…

"Many people, after cancer treatment, long to go back to their normal lives, but there is no going back. What you find instead is a 'new normal.' Take your time; go at a turtle's pace to discover your new normal."

When all of this started, I couldn't wait to get through the treatments so I could get back to my regularly scheduled life. Right. My regularly scheduled life, as my son, Alex, says, "left the building" on October 5, 2010. And there is no going back. And to my surprise, I don't want to go back.

The "new normal" is the perfect description of life after a cancer diagnosis and treatment. My family and I talk about what we'll do in the new normal. Which is great, because the new normal is not just about me, it's about us and the life we create together.

The new normal is What I Leave Behind.
I am leaving behind…

> petty disagreements
> keeping my thoughts and feelings to myself
> unhealthy habits
> the idea that I'll live forever

doing things out of guilt of resentment
rushing around
worries
always putting others' needs before mine

The new normal is What I Find Along the Way. I have found...

a new ability to communicate with the people I love
time to enjoy and soak in nature
strength I didn't know I had
I can trust my instincts
so many people who love and pray for me
patience
I can't force life to go the way I want it to—and that's ok
my priorities have changed

The new normal is What I Intentionally Include. I am intentionally including...

time with family and friends
healthy food that's delicious
exercise and movement of all kinds
time spent outdoors
meditation
crafts I enjoy
thankfulness
joy
doing things out of love and celebration
time to find my passion
a way to give back

I know as time goes on, my family and I will gradually discover and create our new normal. Each day will be a gift we can enjoy together. This experience has changed us all.

Lighthouse
Week 27

This charm was chosen by my mom.
Why? "You are a light to others."

Have you ever had the power go out at night? You understand what pitch black means. And then you light a candle. One tiny candle that seems so insignificant when the lights are on now appears positively radiant in the darkness. It's funny how we notice the light more when there is darkness. When the power goes out, and we're sitting in the dark, we realize how much we take the light for granted, how much we count on instant illumination. When the power's out, and we're relying on candles or flashlights, life slows down. We can't move as quickly as we'd like. We can't see everything at once. There's more mystery as our surroundings are illuminated a bit at a time. And a single candle seems so very bright, drawing our attention.

A power outage is a bit like being diagnosed with cancer. It's as if all the lights went off, and you're now sitting in the dark. You're feeling anxious and alone. You're wondering what's going to happen. You're hoping that someone made a terrible mistake. It feels like the dark is everywhere. It feels like you may never see light again. You will, I promise, but before you do, try this. Give yourself permission to sit in the dark. Allow yourself to feel scared and lonely, confused and angry, overwhelmed and anxious. Once you've permitted yourself to feel all of the emotions a cancer diagnosis brings, you can release them, let them go. And when you do, it's time to leave the dark and find your light.

You may discover that your light is like a starry night, with pinpoints of brightness sparkling in the sky. Or perhaps you will find that your light is like the full moon, illuminating the night with a soft glow. Your light may appear slowly, the way a sunrise does, one ray at a time. Or perhaps you'll find your light in several places at once, like candles flickering around the room. You may find that your light is bright and sudden, as if someone flipped on a spotlight. No matter what your light looks like, follow it. Leave the darkness behind and live in your light.

Live in the light of LOVE,
And light the world with your heart.

Live in the light of JOY,
And let the light in you shine for others.

Live in the light of HOPE,
And look for light wherever you are.

Live in the light of LIFE,
And choose to live your life in light.

—Gayle Bittinger

Castle
Week 28

This charm was chosen by Auntie Margaret, friend and honorary aunt to Katie and Alex. Why? "You are returning from your crusades in Spokane to your castle, your home."

"Be grateful for the home you have, knowing that at
this moment, all you have is all you need."
—Sarah Ban Breathnach

This summer I felt a little like Dorothy in the movie *The Wizard of Oz*, chanting, "There's no place like home, there's no place like home." If only I'd had those ruby slippers, I could have clicked myself to Spokane and back in a jiffy. But there I go again, wanting to skip parts, to fast forward to the next thing. I have to constantly remind myself that all of this—life, cancer treatments, relationships, everything—is a journey. Trust my journey. Find joy in my journey. Stop and smell the roses on my journey. Be present on my journey. My time in Spokane was a journey, not only in miles traveled, but also in growth—my personal growth.

One of the ways I've grown this summer is to be more intentional about being in the moment… being in this moment. In this moment, I'm ok. I have what I need. I am blessed with more than I could possibly imagine. I am so thankful for the home I have. And my home is so much more than the physical building. It's the love my family and I have for each other, the way we care for and support each other; the way we talk and laugh and cry and sing together. It's cooking together, gardening, baking, playing games, walking, traveling, just hanging out together. Home is a feeling. Home is wherever we are.

Home can be a hotel room in Spokane, Katie's college apartment, a table at a local coffee store, a cabin in the woods, a picnic table at the park.

When I truly believe I have what I need, I am wealthy beyond measure. I can stop striving to be something or someone else. I understand that anything I might wish for, I already have. Like Dorothy in Oz—she always had the ability to go home, she just didn't realize it. I have so much inside of me, I don't need to be constantly striving to be more or different or better. In this moment, what I have is what I need. In the next moment, I may need something different, but it doesn't matter because the next moment is not now.

It's an interesting change in my frame of reference. For most of my life, I've gone through my days making lists of what I need to do, need to buy, need to accomplish. I start with what I need—what I'm lacking—and look for that. I might spend a lifetime looking for that thing I feel I lack. I tell myself, "When I get that one thing, I'll have it all." That sense of satisfaction, of fulfillment, is always in the future.

However, when I start with the idea that I already have what I need, everything changes. There's no more searching and wishing, no more feeling inadequate or waiting for the perfect time. When I know with all of my heart that all I have is all I need, I am free. I am safe. I am home.

When you truly believe you have what you need...

It means you have all the

Time and money, talent and skills, love and friendship,

Joy and passion, vocation and faith

You need.

—Gayle Bittinger

Celtic Heart

Week 29

This charm was chosen by Beth, my massage therapist. Why? "Your journey interconnects us all with love."

This experience has certainly been a journey for me, and there have been so many people involved. It's comforting to think they are all interconnected now because they have chosen to walk with me on this path—helping me, supporting me, and loving me on my journey to healing and wholeness.

The Celtic knot is believed to be a symbol of the crossings of the physical and spiritual paths in our lives and of feelings of everlasting love and interconnectedness. It is such an appropriate symbol for my journey. The past twelve months have been a story of connections for me. How many times did my path cross with just the right person at just the right time? When I was feeling discouraged, my path would cross with someone who would lift me up. When I wasn't sure which way to turn, the insight I needed would be just around the next corner. When I didn't know if I could take that next step, someone would be there to carry me for a while. Every day I felt God working in my life through my connections with others. I am so grateful I did not have to travel this path on my own.

There is a new feeling of interconnectedness in my life. As I walk on my path, I see that it is a reflection of my heart. There is a feeling of grace, of being touched by the spirit. There is a sense of joy in the simplest things—a smile from a stranger, the warmth of a sunny day, or a hug from a friend. There is so much love it takes my breath away. There have been so many people, so many crossings. Each person has been a blessing to me. Each crossing has changed me in some way, given me something to take with me. Yes, this is my journey, but it is also a journey of the many people who are walking with me.

I walk in the heart of my life
On a path with no beginning and no ending.
My path crosses yours and
I experience grace,
I share joy,
I reach out in love.
When you cross my path,
You help me see
My walk and my world in a new way.

On my path, every step is mine,
And, yet, it is more than mine.
Every step I take is more because of you.
Every step I take is blessed
With grace and joy and love
Because your path crossed mine.

—Gayle Bittinger

Treasure Chest

This charm was chosen by me.
Why? You never know what treasures life has in
store for you.

"Life is much more manageable when thought of as a
scavenger hunt as opposed to a surprise party."
—Jimmy Buffet

Life as a surprise party is one adrenaline rush after another.
Each event takes the wind out of me, and after the initial fight or flight
response, once my heart stops pounding, I have to decide if the
surprise is good or bad, if it's what I wanted or something I didn't want
at all. Of course, an occasional adrenaline rush isn't bad, but daily, or
even hourly rushes, are a lot to handle. It's stressful on my mind and
body.

But if life is a scavenger hunt, then I never know what treasure
is waiting for me around the corner, behind the door, on the phone, or
in the next moment. It's really a mindset. I see what I'm looking for. If
I believe that the things that happen or appear in my life are treasures,
then I see them differently. I may be skeptical at first—having breast
cancer is a treasure? But when I stop seeing it as a terrifying surprise, I
can open my eyes, and my heart, to find the treasure in it.

Have you ever been on a scavenger hunt? You are given a list
of items to find. The items are typically unusual and completely
unrelated (you won't find them all in the same place). You generally
work with a small group of people and a time limit to find as many of
the items as you can. What is so wonderful about a scavenger hunt,
however, is that the treasures you find on your hunt are not just the

---

items on your list. The treasures are the things you experience along the way. It's meeting the neighbor who gives you a string of ten paperclips while her dog plays with you and lets you scratch its stomach. It's the passing motorist who sees you standing on the corner looking confused, stops to ask if you're lost, and then gives you a street map so you can check one more item off your list. A great scavenger hunt is about connections—creating connections with the people in your group, making connections with the people you meet, connecting everyday items to treasures.

My journey with breast cancer has been a scavenger hunt of the most extraordinary kind. I have found treasures in unexpected places and with unexpected people. My journey has been blessed with so many treasures. It has made me want to be more intentional about being a treasure in other people's lives. As I meet people in my daily life, I ask myself, "How can I be a treasure to this person right now?" It could be a smile, a conversation, a letter, a batch of cookies, a handshake, or a hug. Whatever it is, I can choose to be a treasure to the people in my life every day.

Life as a scavenger hunt is

Unwrapping presents all day long,

Looking for the treasure in every moment,

Putting on your adventurer's hat,

Embracing whatever comes your way,

And finding treasure in unexpected places.

—Gayle Bittinger

Faith-Hope-Love

This charm was chosen by John, the love of my life and husband of 28 years. Why? "Faith, hope, and love, and the greatest of these is... hope."

Being diagnosed with cancer feels like a betrayal. It's tempting to want to climb under the covers and stay there. Or to think that maybe you can avoid it, maybe it won't be real, maybe it will go away if you don't talk about it. Reaching out to my family and friends was one of the hardest things I've ever done. I knew telling them would make them cry, and I didn't want to be the reason for their tears.

Yet, as difficult as it was, when I was finally able to reach out to family and friends, the fear of the unknown, the anxiety about what might happen, the worry of how I would handle treatment—all of that disappeared. When I allowed them into my weak and vulnerable spots, the fear, anxiety, and worry no longer had a place to hide. Reaching out is what has made this journey bearable for me, knowing that my friends and family "have my back," like it says on my son, Alex's, T-shirt.

The support of my family and friends reminds me of a spider web. Each strand is essential to the structure and purpose of the web. Have you ever watched a spider spin a web? To start, she climbs to a chosen starting point and casts a thread into the air, waiting for it to catch on something suitable. Once it does, she can step out onto the thread and begin to create the frame of her web. You'll notice that she can't start building her web until she takes that first risk—casting her thread into the air. It reminds me of those first phone calls I made, the first email I sent to friends and family, telling them I had breast cancer. I was scared, uncertain. I didn't know what to expect. But once I tossed that first strand into the air, I was able to begin building my web of support, strand by strand, email by email, card by card, prayer by prayer.

It became clear that I couldn't do this alone. The more support I had, the stronger my web got. It was easy to see that a web with one or two strands wouldn't be able to catch anything, but a web with dozens of strands could catch a feast. And catch a feast I did, one I could not have imagined, one I could have caught only by taking a risk and casting out that first thread. And like a spider's web, it is the many strands that make me strong, give me courage, and show me the way to healing and wholeness. It is the way my web is constructed with anchors and frames and spirals that helps it stand up to predators and stormy weather. It is all the parts working together that set the stage for a feast of faith and love and hope.

Apple
Week 32

"If you want to make an apple pie from scratch, you must first create the universe." —Carl Sagan

I love the way this quote takes what I think I know—how to make an apple pie from scratch—and turns it upside down. It changes my perspective, the way being diagnosed with cancer changed my idea of what's important and what's not.

What's Important

people
time to connect
doing what's meaningful to me
taking care of myself
acknowledging my feelings

What's Not

things
rushing around doing as much as possible
impressing the neighbors
putting everyone else's needs above mine
pretending

What's important—having no evidence of disease. What's not important—needing to be symptom free right now. It all comes back to patience and being in the moment. I am struggling with this in-between time. Treatments are mostly done, except for Herceptin infusions every other week, and one more surgery next spring. But I'm not feeling 100 percent. It's harder almost than being in active treatment. I'm having a difficult time adjusting to my new normal. What do I do now? How do I see my life differently? Besides a breast cancer survivor, what do I want to be when I grow up?

> "Anyone can count the seeds in an apple, but only God
> can count the number of apples in a seed."
> —Robert H. Schuller

God knows my hopes and fears, my struggles and imperfections. And God loves me. It inspires me to think that God can look at me and see all of my potential, the "number of apples in me," so to speak. I find myself wondering what my potential is. What is it I'm meant to do? Why am I here? Those are big questions with small, doable answers. I want them to be big, amazing answers. I want them to be spectacular, noteworthy answers. But that's not how an apple begins, and that's not how the answers begin. The answers begin with the small stuff, with what I do today. The answers begin with taking that first step, then the next one, and the one after that. The answers begin with a smile on my face and hope in my heart, and the love and grace of God enfolding me.

Let go and let God…
Work in your life, be present in your life,
Bless your life, give you grace,
Grant you peace, and fill your heart with love.

—Gayle Bittinger

High-Heeled Shoe

Week 33

This charm was chosen by Dr. Evans, my breast surgeon. Why? I'm not entirely certain, but it does remind me of her, as does the saying below.

"Today… Be Blessed, Be Strong, Be Beautiful,
Be You!"—Author Unknown

Today… Be Blessed

The best way to be blessed is to open my eyes and heart and count my blessings. If I want to be blessed, I can start with being grateful. When I am aware of and thankful for the many gifts in my life, I can't help but feel blessed.

Today… Be Strong

I had no idea I could be so strong. I always thought it would be terrible to lose my hair. I miss my hair, but it's not terrible to be without it. I love my wig, which helps. I wasn't sure I'd be strong enough to get through a bilateral mastectomy. I wasn't—by myself. I was, with the help of my husband, John. (It just says, "Be strong." It doesn't say I have to be strong all by myself.) I've learned that being strong means taking baby steps, sometimes baby, baby steps. I've learned that being strong means I ask for help when I need it. And I've learned that being strong means acknowledging my fears, worries, and anxieties, and then letting them go.

Today… Be Beautiful

It's hard to feel beautiful with a fuzzy bald head, nausea, mouth sores, and a chemo tan. I love the moments when John holds me and rubs my bald head and tells me I'm beautiful. When he says it, I can mostly believe it. And whenever I look in the mirror, I try to see myself through his eyes, through his love.

I also choose to wear a wig and breast prostheses. I feel more like myself. And for me, that's the key to feeling, being beautiful. I like doing whatever it takes to help me feel like me. Not to cover up or hide or deny what's going on, but to find myself in all of the treatments and the side effects, to be beautiful.

Today... Be You

Today, I can be me, a person with hopes and fears, dreams and wishes, a person who feels love, hope, anger, frustration, anxiety, joy, happiness, excitement. Maybe having cancer makes that one the easiest of all because I just don't have time for nonsense. I don't have time for pretending. I just have time to be myself—blessed, strong, and beautiful.

If you want to be blessed,

Fill your life with gratitude.

If you want to be strong,

Realize you don't have to do it alone.

If you want to be beautiful,

Look at yourself through the eyes of love.

If you want to be you,

Just be yourself.

Today. Right now. This moment.

—*Gayle Bittinger*

Sunflower

This charm was chosen by me, thinking about my beautiful and sunny daughter, Katie. Why? Sunflowers are bright and happy. All it takes to grow a big, gorgeous sunflower is one small seed.

"Walk toward the sunshine and the shadows will always fall behind you." —Mary Engelbreit

Walk toward the sunshine, the light, the warmth, the rays, the glowing orb of plasma. Why would anyone choose to walk in any other direction? I imagine I am standing at an intersection. I look to my left. It's dark and stormy. I see big thunderclouds. There's an ominous feeling, a sense of fear and uncertainty. I see the streaks of rain and sleet, hear the distant thunder, glimpse the flashes of far-off lightning. It's scary.

Now I look to my right. The sky is bright blue and clear. I see the snow-capped mountains glistening in the sunshine. I feel the warmth. I hear birds chirping. Flowers are blooming, lifting their heads to the light. A stream ripples nearby, cascading over rocks.

It's my choice. Will I walk towards the shadows and darkness or walk towards the warm, bright sunshine. It seems obvious, doesn't it? Of course I would choose to walk towards the sunshine. And yet, how often do I choose to walk towards the shadows?

I choose shadows when I...

focus on what I don't have
allow anger and fear to dictate my life
keep my heart closed
put busyness ahead of people
count possessions instead of blessings
live in the past or long for the future
spend time judging instead of loving

I choose sunshine when I...

count my blessings
live in joy and celebration
practice *ephphatha*—openness
reach out
spend time with the people in my life
be present in the moment
love unconditionally

Of course, it could be said that if I just looked to the sunshine, I'd be missing reality, and I would agree. There will always be shadows—cancer, illness, loss, financial troubles, fear, anger—they are a part of life. The choice becomes about where my heart lives, in sunshine or in shadows, because joy, happiness, blessings, love, and grace—they are also a part of life.

Walk towards the sunshine...

If I could only remember to take my own advice! Yesterday, I had a mostly miserable day. I can even pinpoint the exact moment when I was at the intersection of sunshine and shadows and chose to start walking into the darkness. It's a little scary to think I could so completely embrace the shadows. So the question becomes, what do I do when I realize I've taken a wrong turn?

First of all, I must recognize that I've made a wrong turn—warning signs that I've veered into the storm, such as uttering any sentence that begins with "I never" or "I always," feeling afraid, wanting to give up or run away, being indecisive, moping. Once I recognize the warning signs, I can choose to turn toward the sunshine. I can stop. Breathe. Ask for a hug. Let people know what I'm feeling. Count my blessings. Look for possibilities. Call a friend. Do something for me. Take a nap. Help someone. It's never too late to choose to walk towards the sunshine.

Cross
Week 35

*This charm was chosen by me.
Why? I am grateful for a trip taken to a
monastery years ago.*

When I was first diagnosed with cancer, I felt like I had been slapped in the face. It was such a shock. I started thinking about the big why… "Why me?" I was told by some that it was all part of God's plan for me, which just brought me back to the first question—why me? Was it hereditary? Was it environmental? Was it something I did or something I didn't do? There was a tiny part of me that was mad at God, wondering why He would let this happen to me.

Then something happened. I'm not entirely sure what. Maybe it was the softening and letting go of my emotions that happens when I meditate. Maybe it was the prayers of family and friends. I feel like the ice has melted, the dam has broken, that my heart has grown two sizes too big. I feel relief. I feel a soul change. Maybe it was because of the prayer beads.

Many years ago, my husband, daughter, dad, and I took a trip to an Episcopalian monastery on Guemes Island in Washington state's San Juan Islands. At the monastery, we had the opportunity to walk a labyrinth and to make prayer beads. It was a great experience. We had fun spending time together, but I don't think any of us ever imagined the ripples that one trip would create in our lives.

One of the things I have been practicing this year is to act on my hunches. Instead of talking myself out of them, instead of waiting until tomorrow, I've been choosing to act. And the results have been amazing. It feels like I'm passing God's love along, and as it passes through me, I experience it in a way I haven't felt for a while. And the focus changes from me and what's happening to me, to you and ways I can reach out to you, care for you, love you. "I wonder how Laurie K. is doing?" Call her. "That's a great card for LaLani." Send it. "John would love that." Pick it up for him. "Katie had a test today. I wonder how it went." Text her. "I wonder if Alex would like to play cribbage." Ask him. "I would like to give my counselor, Tess, some prayer beads." Make a set for her.

I'm discovering that you never know where the ripples of a small act of kindness will take you. When I made the prayer beads to give to Tess, I didn't even know for sure if she would like them. I knew she'd be polite, and she'd appreciate the fact that I'd made them for her. What I didn't know was that she uses prayer beads regularly and had recently given her only set to a friend in need. I'm so glad I followed my hunch.

As we were talking about the beads and how I had made them, Tess commented that many of the people she works with would love prayer beads. That was it: the spark, a way to give back. My family and I made a dozen sets for Tess to give to her patients and students. She loved them. They loved them. So we've made more. It has become our prayer bead ministry. Sphere of Hope is what John calls it—a Sphere of Hope for me, for us, for fellow cancer patients, for everyone—a ripple of hope and love, faith and peace from a trip taken years ago.

May you find hope in a touch, a glance, a word.

May love greet you at the door and invite you in.

May faith gently encourage and support you.

May peace envelop you and fill your spirit.

—*Gayle Bittinger*

Cupcake
Week 36

This charm was chosen by my friend Margaret D. Why? "Because cupcakes are upbeat and resilient."

Margaret writes…

"Upbeat and happy—Cupcakes are cheerful, full of wonderful tastes, great colors, and decorated individually to anyone's taste. For me, that represents you. No matter what the challenge, you decorate your life with happiness, adjusting to the ebb and flow so that you remain as upbeat as possible. You seem to decorate your life with people, activities,… and charms that reflect what you want life to be—not what you are coping with.

"Resilient—Cupcakes are resilient. They manage to make it to every classroom birthday party. Even if the child drops the pan on the sidewalk, the cupcake papers keep the little morsels intact. All you have to do is scrape the icing off the lid of the pan. You are resilient. This has been a long journey. You 'fall' on the floor, but get back up. Your family protects you, but ultimately it is your resilience that enables you to scrape the icing and goodies off the disappointments and turn them into treats."

A cupcake is a celebration, a party, an event, a gala. It's like someone made a cake just for you. You could have a cupcake every day because there is something to celebrate every day. What was your "cupcake moment" today? It could be something you did for someone else. It could be something someone did for you. It might be time spent with someone special. Perhaps it was an unexpected phone call or letter or package. It could be a rousing game of Ping Pong after dinner. Maybe it was those ten minutes all to yourself in your favorite chair. Cupcake Moments are everywhere, once you start looking for them.

Once you've identified your Cupcake Moment, then it's time to choose the cupcake you would make to commemorate it. Was your moment a Double Fudge Cupcake Moment? Or perhaps it would best be remembered as a Spice Cake With Maple Frosting Moment? Or was it a Cherry Chip With Vanilla Frosting and a Cherry on Top Cupcake Moment? Would your cupcake have a filling? Fruity or creamy? Would it have nuts or sprinkles or chocolate chips?

I can think of several Cupcake Moments I've had lately. Today was the Chocolate With Mocha Frosting Topped With Chocolate-Covered Espresso Beans Cupcake Moment when I surprised John at work with his favorite coffee drink. Yesterday afternoon, my son, Alex, asked if I'd like to watch a favorite show with him. I'd call that a Rainbow Chip With Chocolate Ganache Filling and Whipped Cream Frosting Cupcake Moment. And that surprise phone call from my graduate-school daughter, Katie, was most definitely a Sunny Lemon With Lemon Curd Filling and Devonshire Cream Frosting Cupcake Moment. Delivering a batch of cupcakes to the staff and patients at Columbia Basin Hematology and Oncology with my family was a Raspberry Swirl With Creamy Almond Frosting and Sprinkles Cupcake Moment—and lots and lots of fun.

There are Cupcake Moments happening every day, just look around. And if one can't be found, create one! Make it a point to celebrate a Cupcake Moment every day, and every now and then, whip up a batch of cupcakes to share!

Purse

This charm was chosen by me.
Why? I choose what I carry around with me, and
I want to choose more carefully.

I sit here wondering where my week took a wrong turn—again! It really is a combination of things—the underlying anxiety of being treated for breast cancer, no estrogen (PMS anyone?), a few old aches and pains, being tired, and feeling like I have too much to do. But I want to lighten my heart. I want to live in the moment, to live in a story of hope and joy and love.

So this week, the question is, what do I want to carry in my purse of life? What do I need? What can I leave behind? My real purse used to be pretty heavy. I hauled just about everything in it, until back and neck pain forced me to make a choice—take pain medication on a regular basis or lighten my load. So I lightened my load, tossed out a few things, eliminated duplicates, simplified. And it worked pretty well. Occasionally, I didn't have something I thought I needed, but I either figured out something else or realized I could do without.

And I was doing fine with my lighter purse, until I was diagnosed with breast cancer and had a bilateral mastectomy. Now I have to be very careful about weight on my shoulders. It was time to go through my purse again. I thought I had it down to bare necessities before, but I needed to shed even more. It's amazing how much I had that I believed was necessary, how many trappings and things I had collected. Now my purse is light and has very few things in it. I carry just what is absolutely necessary, which is less than I thought. It's so easy to carry now. I wear it across my body, and my hands are free.

That is a very interesting metaphor for life… am I living a hands-free life? Or am I hanging onto so much baggage that my hands are full, and I can't manage anything else? I can't reach out to help; I can't hold a friend's hand or share a hug. Is my mind so full of how to manage everything that there's no space for anything else? Am I living a hands-free life? Are my hands and heart and mind open and free to experience life, right now, in this moment?

What will I keep in the purse of my hands-free life?

gratitude for my many, many blessings
love given and love received
kindness to myself and others
hope in all things
faith in the God who is with me always

What will I leave behind?

pain from hurts long ago
guilt for being true to myself
fear of not being loved for who I truly am
time spent wishing things were different

I am choosing a heart that is light and full of love. I am choosing a life that is free to be in the moment, to be present, to be now. I am choosing a hands-free life.

Ladybug
Week 38

This charm was chosen by Bobbie, my chemotherapy scheduler at Columbia Basin Hematology and Oncology. Why? "For our Katiebug Ladybug daughters."

How to Get Through Life
"Sleep as much as you can.
Read books you enjoy.
Play with simple things.
Look for affection when you need it.
Get serious once in a while.
Forget about diets.
Show some affection.
Get angry once in a while.
Change your looks.
Above all, be happy
Regardless of what your challenges may be."
—Author Unknown

My dear friend Cyndi sent this poem to me. It's great advice for anyone, but especially for someone going through what I call a "life-altering illness." And having breast cancer is nothing if not life-altering. I'm only beginning to realize how much. Thinking about the new normal helps, but it doesn't accurately depict the enormity of the whole process. So here's my version of "How to Get Through Life" for the new normal.

How to Live in the New Normal

Rest and take care of yourself—
You think you can go full speed, but you can't, not yet.

Do things you enjoy—
Without guilt and with joy and celebration.

You do not need to make things complicated.
Play, work, live with simplicity.

You have so many people who love you
and want to be there for you.

Some things just need to be done (laundry, dishes).
Do them in small chunks, so you won't get overwhelmed.

Your body knows what it wants to eat.
And remember, chocolate comes from the fruit of the cacao tree.

Reach out. Help someone else.
Make face-to-face connections.

Your feelings are your feelings.
Acknowledge them and then let them go.

It's just hair—real hair, wig hair, no hair.
It's your choice.

There is always joy to be found, just look around.

—Gayle Bittinger

The new normal is difficult. I thought I was ready for it, but it's so much more challenging than I anticipated. And yet, I still come back to the idea that my life now, my new normal, is richer and fuller and more satisfying than ever. "There is always joy to be found, just look around."

Paper Airplane
Week 39

This charm was chosen by me.
Why? It reminds me of my son, Alex, making
paper airplanes by the dozens as he explored the
science of flight, precision folding, and going
with the flow.

When I want to learn to do something well, it helps if I am persistent enough to practice, persnickety enough to pay attention to the details, and personable enough to work well with others. Practicing those three characteristics is also a great way for me to thrive in the new normal.

Persistent

Being persistent is essential in the new normal. Consistency, for me, is the key to feeling my best. Doing the things that help me heal and keep me emotionally and physically healthy is so important. When I'm persistent, I feel so much better. But it's hard. And most of the difficulties or opposition comes from myself. I've never been able to stick to an exercise routine for any length of time—until now. I feel so much better when I exercise and walk once or twice a day. But sometimes I just want to sit around and watch TV or read a book or bake cookies, and the time for exercising slips away. I must be persistent in doing the things that help me feel my best because then I'll have the time and strength to do the other things I'd like to do.

Being persistent also means following my instincts, listening to my gut, doing what I know is the best for me. There are many people who are happy to offer advice, and I have to figure out what suits me—what works for me, regardless of what others do or say. For me, being persistent plays a key in helping me feel my best.

Persnickety

Hmm… a seemingly negative quality, and it could easily become annoying and exhausting, but paying attention to details makes the new normal even better. I pay a lot more attention to the little things that bring joy into my life. I try to spend less time rushing from one thing to the next and more time enjoying the details of my life. It's the little things that make life so much richer—candles lit for dinner, a clean kitchen counter, a neat and tidy craft room, getting dressed in the morning, making my family's favorite cookies. Of course, it's possible to take the details too far and miss out on living life, but spending a little time to make something extra special (not perfect, just special) is worth the effort. It's knowing how to balance the big and little details of my life that makes the difference.

Personable

My plan to Kick Some Cancer Butt was to gather my team and work together. I wanted providers who would work with me, explain treatments to me, answer all of my (many!) questions, and allow me to be involved in my healing. And being personable makes that so much easier—on all sides. Working with providers who are caring and personable as well as being involved and personable myself are key. It's funny. A diagnosis of cancer could have made me angry, depressed, and anxious—and it did, for a while. Mostly, though, it made me realize that I didn't want to spend a lot of time feeling angry, depressed, or anxious. Life's too short to spend my time that way. I prefer to spend my time greeting each day in a pleasant manner, offering a smile to everyone I meet, letting the little things go, in short, having a pleasant appearance and manner each day because being personable is the best possible choice.

Rainbow & Cloud

Week 40

This charm was chosen by Dr. Rado, my oncologist at Columbia Basin Hematology and Oncology. Why? He considered the compass, then chose this one. (I forgot to ask why.)

It's funny that I picked up this charm just last week. It spoke to me, too. Bright and happy, with a colorful rainbow and a cloud. That's life—rainbows and clouds—and learning how to live in love and joy, even when a storm arrives.

It takes rain and sunshine to make a rainbow, and the only way I can see a rainbow is to stand with my back to the sun, looking into the rain. It's scary to look into my "rain"—those feelings of fear, pain, guilt, and resentment in my life—but when the sun is at my back, when I know there is light and life waiting for me, looking at the rain reveals a brilliant rainbow, a rainbow that conveys a promise of hope and love and the knowledge that my journey is to be trusted.

When John and I first met with Dr. Rado, we were more than a little overwhelmed—chemo, surgery, chemo, radiation, a year of biotherapy, and a surgery for risk reduction, whew! At every appointment, I was healthy enough to receive the next treatment. I was thankful for that at the time, but I am especially thankful now that I understand it doesn't always work that way. Sometimes your body isn't strong enough to withstand the treatment. Sometimes you're healthy enough, but the treatment is unavailable. I don't know how I would have felt if I couldn't have had my scheduled treatments. Being healthy enough to be treated and having those treatments available is what I call a "rainbow blessing."

A Rainbow Blessing is something that happens when I find myself in the middle of a storm. My past year has been filled with grace and blessings that would have never happened if I hadn't been diagnosed with breast cancer.

My diagnosis of breast cancer, a storm of enormous proportions, has brought so many blessings into my life—the people I've met and gotten to know along the way, the time to sort out what is truly important to me, and the courage to try new things. But the biggest blessing—understanding and knowing in my heart how very blessed I am every moment of every day—is the best Rainbow Blessing of all.

"Life isn't about waiting for the storm to pass…
It's learning to dance in the rain."—Anonymous

There will always be storms. That's life. The question is what will I do with the storms in my life? Will I hunker down, with my back to the storm, closed off from the world, waiting for the rain to stop? I could be in for a long wait, and in the process, I've closed myself off to everything and everyone, not just the storm. I can't see the rainbow if I'm hiding under my umbrella.

Or when the storm arrives, will I look for the rainbow while I'm dancing in the rain? Will I take in the dazzling colors while I get soaking wet? Will I get up and dance and celebrate life in all of its imperfections? The only way to see the rainbow is to step out into the rain.

Cinderella
Week 41

This charm was chosen by me.
Why? The impossible can happen every day.

"Once in a while... right in the middle of an ordinary life... Life gives you a Fairy Tale." —Author Unknown

Does it seem strange to be writing about fairy tales after a cancer diagnosis? Before my diagnosis, I would have said, "What in the world are you thinking?" A year later, it seems perfectly natural. What is a fairy tale? It is a story that features a fair maiden (that would be me); a mean, rotten, nasty, scary antagonist (a dragon or, perhaps, an evil step-mother, although in this case, that would be my diagnosis of breast cancer), and a handsome prince (that would be my husband, John).

"Once upon a time, John and I had a very nice, very normal life—going along our way, raising two wonderful children, celebrating our 27th wedding anniversary, just happy being together. When, out of the blue, a diagnosis of breast cancer landed in my life. I felt like Snow White when she was tossed into the scary forest. There were so many things coming at me. I didn't know what they were. I didn't know what to do. I couldn't see the path just yet, and I was frightened.

"But then, my prince arrived, and, to be honest, he was scared, too. But he wrapped his arms around me and held me and shared his strength and peace and faith with me. Then, together we went out and slayed the dragon and lived happily ever after. The end."

This fairy tale that started with a scary, breath-taking diagnosis of breast cancer has catapulted John and me into a place of love and delight and appreciation, into a life of awareness and gratitude and celebration. It is a fairy tale with a happily ever after that we experience each moment we're together.

"I have found the one whom my soul loves."
—Song of Solomon 3:4

That's how I know things are the way they are supposed to be. It feels right in my soul. Sometimes I don't know why things are happening the way they are, where the twists and turns of my life are leading me, and then all of a sudden I turn a corner and realize, "This is why I'm here." It reminds me of a hike John and I took to a hidden lake off the Mountain Loop Highway in Snohomish County, Washington. After hiking up the mountainside for what seemed like hours, I was certain we had missed a turn somewhere. John suggested we hike one more switchback. We did, and as we turned the corner— there was the lake: gorgeous and blue, tucked into the side of Mt. Pilchuck. The photograph John took of this lake is hanging in our bedroom. It reminds me to trust that my life is leading me in the direction I am meant to go and that each step I take is the one I am meant to take.

I have found

The one whom my soul loves,

The life I am meant to live,

The path I am meant to travel,

And my heart in all that I do.

—Gayle Bittinger

Shooting Stars

This charm was chosen by me.
Why? My family and I love to go outside on a
summer night and look at the stars. We especially
enjoy August nights during the Perseid Meteor
Showers when we watch for shooting stars.

"Before the big bang, before time itself, before matter, energy, velocity; there existed a single immeasurable state called yearning. This is the special force that on a day before there were days obliterated nothing into everything. It is the unseen strings tying planets to stars. It is the maddening want we feel from first breath to last light."
—Mary Shannon (From the TV show, *In Plain Sight*)

I believe this yearning is love: wanting to love and be loved, to be connected to one another, to be in relationship. It was love, God's love, that obliterated nothing into everything. It is love that ties us together—people, families, cities, countries, planets, stars, galaxies. It is love that gets us out of bed in the morning, and it's love that tucks us in at night.

In so many ways, this past year has been a story of love. I've felt scared, lonely, angry, worried, terrified, anxious, aggravated, frustrated, nervous (the list could go on). But those feelings were transient. The only feeling that has truly been a constant is love—the love of my family and friends, the love shown by neighbors, acquaintances, and strangers, God loving and caring for me in more ways and through more people than I could have ever imagined.

I enjoy stargazing with my husband, John. It's something we've done together for decades. Stargazing is part knowledge, part imagination, (those seven stars are a bull?), part awareness of the vastness of this world in which we live. It's difficult to look at the stars without a sense of awe and wonder.

As the Christmas season draws near, I find myself thinking about the three wise men who followed a star to find the babe in the manger. Their intimate knowledge of the skies made it possible for them to recognize a new and important star. But to leave everything and follow it to the new king, that's the real story. They put aside their daily work and traveled thousands of miles (on camels!) to find and worship the king. That was a journey of faith and trust, a belief in something bigger than themselves.

I can relate to their journey, just a little. It started when I noticed something different happening with my body. I consulted with experts. I understood what I needed to do. And then I had to trust. I had to let go of the reins and be willing to go where the star (my journey) led me. The wise men must have had times when they felt discouraged, times when the clouds covered the night sky and their direction seemed unclear. They must have relied on the kindness of the people they met along the way. And then, suddenly, their journey was over. They found the babe, the newborn king, and worshipped him.

And then they returned home by another way. I think that might just be a different way of saying that after their journey, they would never be the same. Because they journeyed to experience God's love in a baby, they would now be traveling and living in a "new normal." I know what that is like. As I've traveled along my journey to healing and wholeness, I know that I will never be the same. Having experienced love and grace and blessings along the way, my world and my life are changed. From now on, I will forever be walking another way, aware of—and thankful for—each moment.

Sun

This charm was chosen by me.
Why? Each day is a new possibility, a chance to
live in the moment, an opportunity to love and
be loved.

"To live is so startling it leaves little time for anything
else."—Emily Dickinson

If I do it right, that is! Each moment is a miracle, a gift from
God. When I recognize that, I start living in the here and now, with no
time for regrets of the past or worries of the future. When I live in the
moment, there is no other time, there is only now. And when I figure
out how to do that, life becomes startling, amazing, and joy-filled.
When my mind gets so full of worries, regrets, and things I want to do,
it becomes a whirlwind of noise and confusion in my head—a
cacophony of distraction. But when I bring myself back to the
moment—back to living—the background noise fades, and I have the
opportunity to be awed and blessed by being in this moment, right
here, right now.

"Dwell in possibilities."—Emily Dickinson

How many of us have an inner "Eeyore" providing color
commentary on our lives? "It will never work." "Might as well try,
there's nothing better to do." "No one will notice anyway." I feel sorry
for Eeyore; life never seems to go right for him. But then, life rarely
goes right for Winnie-the-Pooh either. Remember the times he was
chased by bees, stuck in a rabbit hole, or lost in the woods? So why do

I think of Pooh as a happy little bear? Pooh lives in possibilities. He sees life as an adventure.

When I dwell in possibilities, I live in hope. I live with a smile on my face. I live in a place where I have choices. And truthfully, no matter what my circumstances, I have choices: to act with integrity or not, to love or not, to be a friend or not, to be kind or not. When I see my life in terms of possibilities, I see an adventure. I see a journey filled with discoveries around each corner. Dwelling in possibilities means saying yes to life, saying yes to the opportunities that come my way.

Life doesn't always go the way I would like it to go, and how I deal with that when it happens is my choice. I can dwell in impossibilities—the things and choices I no longer have, or I can choose to dwell in the possibilities that my life today offers. Each time the sun rises, a new day offers me a new life and new possibilities.

"Forever is composed of nows."—Emily Dickinson

In the continuum of time, there is only now. When I live in the now, I create a life—a "forever"—of depth and meaning. Each "now" is a building block. The life John and I have is strong and sturdy because of all the "nows" we've created together. Being in the moment, being with one another, being present for one another—that's how we build a forever together. Time spent rehashing the past or fretting about the future takes away from the now. Being in the moment requires letting go of old hurts and regrets. It requires quieting our minds and letting go of worries about the future. Being in the moment is about what we see, hear, touch, taste, and feel right now. It's noticing the little things about the people and places in front of us. It's about focusing on the here and now. Building a forever together starts with moments we share now.

Koru & Sun

This charm was chosen by my daughter, Katie.
Why? "It reminds me of the happy, dancing
Kokopelli on Poppa's T-shirt."

The koru (kaw-roo), a symbol of the Maori, shows a fern frond unfurling. It represents new life, peace, spirituality, and awakening, and is a symbol of loving and nurturing relationships. The koru is so appropriate for me at this point in my journey, because it represents...

New Life

I feel like I've been given a chance for a new life—a new normal—filled with the people, activities, and things of my choosing. What will I create? How will I use this past year to influence and inspire what I do? I am looking forward to being done with treatment. And what a perfect time to finish—near the end of winter, as I'm waiting for spring, for new life and new growth.

Peace

Finding peace seems like an impossible task in the middle of a cancer diagnosis, and yet it is so essential. When I allow myself to settle down, when I let go of worry and guilt and anxiety, peace has a chance to sneak into my heart. And when it does, I feel so much better. The sense of calm, the feeling of tranquility—peace—is exactly what I need. Feeling at peace with myself and my cancer means I am able to look beyond the cancer, to look beyond my treatments, to see the blessing of each moment.

Spirituality

I've learned so many things since being diagnosed with cancer. One of the most important has been to remember to step out in faith each day. This is scary. It means letting go of the control I thought I had and letting God lead. It's hard to do. I like thinking I'm in control, even if I'm not. But I know that when I step out in faith, when I rely on a power greater than myself, I allow blessings and miracles to flow through my life.

Awakening

I find myself awakening to new possibilities, thinking about ways to reach out to others. Should I continue with my journaling so I can share my breast cancer experience with others? Is it time to expand our prayer bead ministry to reach more people? How could I help others learn about living with one of the most common side effects of breast cancer treatment, lymphedema? I feel as if I've been hibernating, and now it's time for me to wake up, time for me to discover what's next.

When you hear the words, "You have cancer,"

It feels as if your world has stopped turning,

As if all that you knew to be true has faded away,

Leaving behind only tests and appointments, treatments and procedures.

Then one day you'll find your treatments are over,

And it's time to embrace your new normal,

To find peace in each moment, to step out in faith,

And to awaken to the possibilities waiting for you.

—Gayle Bittinger

Moon

Week 45

*This charm was chosen by me.
Why? There was a gorgeous full moon in the
western sky this morning.*

I love those moments that make me stop and experience a bit of wonder and joy. The moon was absolutely breath-taking this morning—big and bright and full and right in front of me as I was driving the morning carpool to school. Isn't that the way those moments happen? I'm going about my usual routine, and there it appears—a moment of majesty, a glimpse of the divine—what I would call an "Aaah Moment." I wonder how many Aaah Moments I miss as I rush from one thing to the next, too busy to stop or look up from my to-do list?

> "Make space for joy in your life; let it flow through
> you."—Author Unknown

Make space. That's the ultimate secret of a joy-filled life—space. When I rush around, when I feel like there's too much to do, I feel crowded and cramped, and my first response to any interruption is certainly not joy. Annoyance, perhaps, or irritation, or a bit of impatience. It's time to put a stop to that. It's time to make space in my life for joy. As I look back over the last few months, I can see that any time there's a little something "extra" on the calendar—Halloween, Thanksgiving, birthdays, Christmas—I feel crowded. The space disappears. And the joy follows.

Some of it, of course, is treatment related and requires patience more than anything else. But some of it is an annual "tradition," and I would like to add space to these crowded times of the year. Most of the things that make me feel crazy and crowded are things that I know are coming—Christmas is December 25th. It's always been December 25th, no surprises there. So why was I wrapping gifts after church on Christmas Eve? (And not feeling particularly joyful about it!) There's such a fine line between planning ahead and being in the moment, but I think if I do a little bit of planning ahead, it gives me space for joy.

Which makes me think of two kinds of time. Chronos time is the stopwatch by which most of us live. It is our calendars, appointments, and schedules. Khronos is Greek for "time." This is the time that runs the world. It keeps our families and cities and countries running smoothly. Chronos time is the to-do list for daily living. It's necessary, but it can also take over my day, my week, my month, my life. This is why it is so important to leave space for Kairos time. Kairos time is event-centered time, memorable time, a propitious moment for decision or action. Kairos is Greek for "opportunity." When I leave room for Kairos time, I leave room for the unexpected, for moments of grace, for a beautiful moon in the morning sky. With Kairos time, I leave space in my life for joy.

Chronos time ticks away,

Counting seconds, minutes, hours, days.

Marking out time in predictable, regimented ways.

Chronos time means

Cookies baked exactly right,

Appointments kept,

Birthdays remembered.

Chronos time makes kairos time possible.

Kairos time flows along,

Celebrating events big and small.

Creating opportunities for decision and action.

Kairos time means

Being in the moment,

Going where the day leads,

Spending time without clock or agenda.

Kairos time makes chronos time meaningful.

—Gayle Bittinger

Ice Cream Cone
Week 46

This charm was chosen by Jessica, one of my infusion nurses at Columbia Basin Hematology and Oncology. Why? "Because ice cream is awesome!"

"Life is a great big canvas, and you should throw all the paint on it you can."—Danny Kaye

I love the picture this creates in my mind: a big, wall-sized canvas; drop cloths covering the floor and walls so there are no worries about making a mess; buckets of paint in dozens of colors; and cups, scoops, spoons, and brushes of all sizes. Then there's me, in paint-splattered clothes, gleefully scooping up paint and flinging it on the canvas. I can imagine tossing a big cup of red paint up high; splattering blue across the middle; flinging spoonfuls of purple, yellow, green, orange, and indigo at random. A joyful, vibrant, expression of life that is AWESOME!

I'm not talking about perfection here; I'm talking about life—messy, unpredictable, random, surprising life. And the best thing about this mural of life is that there is no way to control it. Sure I can try to aim that cup of blue paint at the center of the canvas, but who knows exactly where it will land? And if I try to control it, I'll go crazy. Letting go of the results is so liberating. When I stop micromanaging every drop of paint, I can relax, step back, and be amazed by the gorgeous mural I am creating. When I am fully involved in the process, the product isn't unimportant, but it becomes secondary. Putting my focus on the journey instead of the destination means I can enjoy all of the fun along the way. I may even discover something entirely unexpected, entirely different, and entirely better.

"Sometimes on the way to what's supposed to happen,
something even better happens."
—Dick Solomon, High Commander
(from the TV show *3rd Rock From the Sun*)

You can't plan life. Oh, there are those of us who try, but the truth is, it just can't be done. Life is messy. Life is a canvas with paint thrown all over it. And the day I truly knew in my heart that life couldn't be planned and organized and ordered to my specifications was the day I finally let go and learned how to live.

It may be a hard sell to convince anyone that what I thought was supposed to happen, "life without cancer," was replaced by something better. But it's true. Life without cancer was replaced by "an opportunity to see life through new eyes and to be open to the moment, the blessings, and the love." The lessons of living in the moment and being open to the awesomeness of life are best learned the "hard way." Some lessons are like that. They must be experienced to be understood. There is a saying by the Chinese philosopher, Confucius, "I hear and I forget. I see and I remember. I do and I understand." After my year of "doing," I now understand.

In cancer, I found life and discovered

The power of the moment,

The joy of saying yes,

The hope in a hello,

The love in a hug,

The spirit in every person,

And the blessing of each day.

—Gayle Bittinger

Topaz

This charm was chosen by my friend Jean.
Why? "What a challenge. It was hard not to
choose the teddy bear, but you are a lot more
than just soft and cuddly. I choose the topaz."

Topaz
When it is yellow, it brings sunshine.
When it is blue, it brings comfort.
When it is red, it brings strength.

You are "bright" like a topaz.
You "glow" like a topaz.
You bring sunshine and comfort to many people.
You are "hard" when you need to be.
You have "inner strength" when you need it.
—Jean Warren

Sunshine

I choose sunshine whenever possible. I look for sunshine wherever I am. Whether it's choosing laughter over tears or basking in the smiles and support from others, sunshine is essential. It shines light into my dark and scary corners, chasing my fears away. Sunshine warms my soul and reminds me to stay on the path of light and love. Sunshine puts a smile on my heart and a spring in my step. Sunshine helps me move forward on my journey through cancer and treatment into healing and wholeness.

Comfort

Whenever I go on a trip, I always pack a few things that will make me feel more comfortable—my pillow, a blanket, a picture of my family. It's been the same with this journey. The evening I was diagnosed, John and I just held one another. It was a comfort of cosmic proportions to know that he was there, that we were going on this journey together. Whenever I put on the beautiful blue topaz necklace he gave me, I know he's with me, even if he isn't right next to me. I find comfort in our family routines: the way we've made it a point to spend time together watching comedies on TV, playing games with made-up rules, going for walks, creating gourmet meals. There is comfort in taking one moment at a time—at being present and engaged in the here and now, where regrets of the past and worries of the future fade away. Comfort is the absolute assurance that there are people who love and care for me and for whom I love and care.

Strength

We are stronger than we think—every single one of us. Most of us aren't challenged in some life-changing way, so we don't realize how strong we actually are. I learned that I had the strength to receive each chemotherapy treatment, knowing that it would make me sick before it made me better. I learned that I had the strength to go through a physically and emotionally difficult surgery. I learned that I could be strong enough to choose what is right for me, to laugh when I want to cry, to get up and enjoy each day to the best of my ability. I learned that I could be strong enough to accept my limitations, to ask for help. And I learned that I could be strong enough to reach out to others, to be vulnerable, to risk sharing my thoughts and feelings.

As I walk the path from breast cancer diagnosis and treatment to healing and wholeness, I know I have found the sunshine, comfort, and strength I will keep with me forever.

Inspire

Week 48

This charm was chosen by Lois, one of my medical assistants at Columbia Basin Hematology and Oncology
Why? "You inspire us every time you come in. You're an inspiration for how to handle adversity."

"Live today…with all your breath, with all your laughter, with all your kindness, with all your heart."
—Author Unknown

Live today…

It's so tempting to rehash yesterday, questioning my decisions, second-guessing my actions. It's easy to doubt myself, especially when it comes to something so new and different, like a cancer diagnosis. Yesterday is a very tempting place to stay, finding someone or something to blame, hoping to figure out how things took such an unexpected turn. But I can't live in yesterday.

Tomorrow is very distracting, too, with its numerous "what ifs." What if the chemo makes me throw up? What if I lose my hair? What if the cancer comes back? What if an alien space craft lands in my backyard? (Just wanted to see if you were paying attention!) I could spend all my time and energy worrying about things that will never happen. But what if that thing I was most afraid of did happen, would I be able to change it by worrying about it? Probably not. (That alien space craft left its home planet light years ago!) So, I step away from the "what could have been," quiet the "what ifs," and center myself in the "what's here now," which is all I have, to be present in this moment, to live today.

With all your breath...

Take a deep breath, and another, and another. Deep breaths help me feel refreshed, relaxed, aware. When I learned how to breathe—deep belly breaths that renewed my body and spirit—I learned how to live in peace and gratitude.

With all your laughter...

Giggle, chuckle, guffaw, snicker, chortle—laugh every day. I can laugh at the joy of a new day. I can laugh when I finish crying. And if a good laugh is hard to come by at the moment, I can find someone who will laugh for me. I'm not really a jokester. When people came up to me and said, "I love your hair," I never whipped off my wig and replied, "Would you like it?" But I never lost my sense of humor. Laughter is a choice. Each day I can choose to laugh or cry. I choose laughter.

With all your kindness...

I have to admit there are days when I feel like snapping at everyone, days when I am tired of being sick and tired and feeling so unlike myself. It's those days when being kind is the most important thing I can do, and the first person I need to show kindness and compassion to is myself. When I treat myself with kindness, it's easier to treat my whole world the same way.

With all your heart...

For me, this journey is all about love: love overcoming fear, love providing hope, love creating joy. Through everything that's happened this past year, there has been love. Each step has been lighter because love was leading the way. It would have been so easy to let fear or guilt or anxiety take over until I found myself groping in the darkness, wondering how I could get so lost. But when I stop and take a deep breath, I find love there, waiting to show me the way, waiting to show me how to live with all my heart.

Teddy Bear
Week 49

*This charm was chosen by my husband, John.
Why? "The bear reminds me of Winnie-the-
Pooh, and Pooh just is."*

"While Eeyore frets and Piglet hesitates and Rabbit
calculates and Owl pontificates, Pooh just is."
—Benjamin Hoff, *The Tao of Pooh*

Pooh just is. A very difficult concept to embrace in our hurry-up, fill-it-up world. Pooh is an expert at being in the moment, being present. I have tried to be like Pooh on my journey, leaving behind the regrets of yesterday and the worries of tomorrow. Today is what I have. And when my focus is on this moment, everything else melts away. Being in the moment is one of the best gifts I can give myself; soaking up the here and now, basking in my life and my blessings.

There are many ways to be distracted from the moment, to be taken away from the here and now. I sometimes find myself fretting like Eeyore, hesitating with Piglet, calculating like Rabbit, or pontificating with Owl. And I have met people along my journey who act like Eeyores, Piglets, Rabbits, and Owls, distracting me from today, distracting me from just being.

"While Eeyore frets..."

Eeyore lives in a constant state of gloominess. Nothing ever goes right for him. He can't actually imagine things going right. He really only feels in sync with his world when things aren't going his way. "It won't work..." "I'll never..." It is very easy to be an Eeyore after a cancer diagnosis. "My life will never be the same." "This is horrible and unfair." "I'll never feel better." "Sure, I'll go into remission, and then it will come back." "I can't face life without (fill-in-the-blank)." There is probably a bit of Eeyore in all of us. The question becomes, do I let Eeyore dictate how I feel and what I do? Or do I politely acknowledge him, and then tell him to take a hike? When I feel like Eeyore, when I feel like the sun will never shine again, I can take a deep breath. I can be present in the moment and remember that Pooh just is.

"...and Piglet hesitates..."

Piglet's hesitation often makes him appear helpless. He's cautious to the point of missing what's right in front of him. He's afraid to make a mistake, to take a chance. I can understand that. I never used to like to make mistakes or take risks, but now I realize that life is too short to hold back out of fear or doubt. When I'm feeling like Piglet, I am at the mercy of my cancer. But I must remember that I am not helpless. I have choices. Perhaps not every choice I'd like (I can't choose to not have cancer), but I can choose how I deal with it. When I feel like Piglet, when I feel helpless, I can take a deep breath. I can be present in the moment and remember that Pooh just is.

"...and Rabbit calculates..."

Rabbit is clever. He is always planning to do something, running around, getting everyone around him into a tizzy. His plans usually don't work out, though. He's either too clever for his own good or not as clever as he thinks. Either way, he usually overacts and overdoes whatever it is he is trying to do. If he would just slow down a bit, maybe stop to ask for help and be willing to admit he doesn't actually know everything, he could really enjoy life. It's so tempting to be like Rabbit after being diagnosed with cancer. I hoped that if I stayed busy enough making plans, doing something, I wouldn't have to think about the cancer. Maybe I could forget I have cancer if I'm too busy with everything else. But being busy, running around like Rabbit, won't make my cancer go away. Those kinds of things are just distractions. They take me away from the moment. They keep me from acknowledging my reality. They keep me from making peace, from allowing grace into my life. When I feel like Rabbit, when I am running around trying to avoid thinking about what is happening, I can take a deep breath. I can be present in the moment and remember that Pooh just is.

"...and Owl pontificates..."

Owl is seemingly super smart. He thinks he has all the answers, even if he has no idea what he's talking about. He has big words for every occasion. He wants everyone to think he knows everything there is to know about the topic at hand. He uses big words to distract and confuse—if others don't understand him, they won't know how smart he is or isn't. After my cancer diagnosis, I wanted ANSWERS. "Why did this happen to me?" "What is it?" "How can I make it go away?" It is so easy to get caught up in the search for knowledge, to spend hours on the Internet looking for answers, to jump on information from the "latest study." There are many Owls out there, distracting me with the "cure of the day." When I feel like Owl, when I want answers and feel frantic to find them, I can take a deep breath. I can be present in the moment and remember that Pooh just is.

"...Pooh just is."

Pooh is a bear who lives in the moment, who understands who he is, and is at peace with that. "I am a bear of very little brain and big words bother me," he tells Owl after listening to one of Owl's monologues. Pooh is just making a statement. Not judging himself, not wishing he was smarter, not even asking Owl to use smaller words. Pooh just is. After a cancer diagnosis, it is so tempting to fret and worry like Eeyore, to feel hesitant and helpless like Piglet, to be clever and calculating like Rabbit, or to hide behind Owl's apparent knowledge, but Pooh has the right approach. Pooh just is.

I am a woman

Who has been diagnosed with breast cancer.

I am seeking

The best possible treatment for my body and mind.

I am being true

To myself in my writing.

I am spending my time in the here and now,

Not rushing around, not searching for whatever I think I might need.

I am trusting

That I am where I am meant to be.

I am living and loving

Each moment I have.

—*Gayle Bittinger*

Silver Heart

Week 50

This charm was chosen by my husband, John, and my son, Alex. Why? "Your last Herceptin treatment is on Valentine's Day."

"A light heart lives long."—William Shakespeare

What does it mean to have a light heart? A light heart is filled with joy. It is not weighted down with regrets and worries, guilt and anger. A light heart is a heart that knows its true path. It doesn't force itself to be something it's not.

A light heart is a wagon with round wheels. Have you ever tried to pull a wagon with square wheels? Of course not, it would be much too difficult, especially since you know that round wheels make pulling a wagon incredibly easy. I imagine I'm pulling a wagon on my journey through life. When I am making choices that feel right, choices that reflect the true me, it feels like my wagon has round wheels. The wagon is easy to pull and the load I'm carrying moves smoothly, even over rough terrain. And, best of all, my heart is light. However, when I am making choices out of guilt or expectations or am doing things that don't resonate with me, my wagon feels as if it has square wheels. And a wagon with square wheels is difficult to pull. Moving it even just a little bit requires so much extra effort.

I know when my wagon has round wheels. My life is flowing. There's no sense of forcing things to work out. I'm not trying to fit square pegs into round holes. I'm not redesigning the square pegs or making the round holes a little bigger. When the wheels are round, life works just as it is. It means that the things I am doing are the things that are truly meaningful to me. And meaningful to me is not the same as "good for me," "educational," "useful," or "expected." It means I am doing what is important to me in a way that works for my life.

For me, pulling a wagon with round wheels—having a light heart—means listening to that voice inside of me. I know when my heart is light and the wheels on my wagon are round. I also know, if I'm honest with myself, when my heart is heavy and the wheels on my wagon are square. And once I understand the difference between living my life with round wheels and living my life with square wheels, I can make choices to include as many round wheels in my life as possible and to just leave the square wheels behind. Going through life with round wheels and a light heart fills my journey with joy and turns it into a celebration.

Square Wheels

cancer research on the Internet
long phone calls
never-ending to-do lists
guilt
obligation
strict schedules
anxiety
what ifs

Round Wheels

providers who patiently explain
letters and cards in my mailbox
to-do lists with three items
gratitude
choice
routines
laughter
being in the moment

Compass

This charm was chosen by Carleen and Emily, baristas at my favorite coffee shop. Why? "Through all of this, you found your own true north."

Finding your way with a compass is a lost art. Today, the thing to use is the Global Positioning System (GPS). According to all the advertisements, I'll never be lost again if I have a GPS—as long as it has power; the locations I'm looking for are in its memory; and the roads it wants me to travel on are not closed for construction, a street festival, or the largest 3-on-3 basketball tournament in the country.

I use a GPS occasionally, but it's not my favorite way to navigate. Whenever I try to alter my course after programming my GPS, "Make the first legal U-turn" or "Recalculating route" is ringing in my ears in no time. And my GPS has very little imagination. It will decide on one or two major thoroughfares in a city, and then direct me to those, regardless of my destination and regardless of whether there is a simpler way to get where I want to go using less traveled roads. A GPS is also not as accurate as it would like me to believe. I was driving on the freeway, but my GPS thought I was on the adjacent side road, traveling well over the speed limit, which it warned me about—repeatedly.

When I chose to have my radiation treatments in Spokane, I knew I'd have to become familiar with driving in a new city. After a week of GPS-directed travel, I decided to set out on my own. I bought an old-fashioned paper map, wrote out general directions to my appointments based on landmarks I knew I could find, and then explored. I was free to discover a new avenue without recalculating my route. I was free to travel the long way or skip to the shortcut. I was free to decide for myself if I was on the freeway or a side road. Once I left the GPS behind, I was free to develop a true sense of the city. Once I stopped relying on another's interpretation of the world around me, I was able to see for myself where I was. I was free to choose my own path.

That's an uncanny analogy for what happened when I was told I had cancer. At first I was scared and overwhelmed, grasping at any information or advice I could find. I was in a new place. I felt lost and more than a little scared. (If you think being lost in a big city is scary, try being lost in the first few days of a cancer diagnosis.) So, in the beginning, I let my GPS (doctors, nurses, family, friends, books, Internet) tell me what to do, and that was ok. I needed time to get a feel for what was happening, to see for myself where I was. But once I knew, it was time to locate my own map, choose my own landmarks, and find my own way. It was time to do the things that made sense to me.

This was when I realized that, while I didn't get to choose whether or not I wanted to take this journey, I did get to choose how I would travel along the way; I was free to choose my own path. And that's what this year-long journey has been for me, an opportunity to find and trust my inner compass, to find my own true north.

When you trust your inner compass,

You explore new paths with courage.

When you trust your inner compass,

You dare to be yourself.

When you trust your inner compass,

You find your own true north.

—Gayle Bittinger

Week 52
Zero

This charm was chosen by my daughter, Katie.
Why? "You have zero treatments left!"

Zero treatments left; I can't believe this day has actually arrived. I knew it would come, of course, but I haven't spent much time thinking about life after treatment. I'm excited and terrified all at the same time.

I really thought this journal entry would be all about the celebrating—zero chemotherapy to go, zero radiation treatments to go, zero Herceptin infusions, zero, zero, zero! But I find myself in an odd place. I'm happy (ecstatic!) that my treatments are over. I'm thrilled to start remembering what my body feels like when it isn't coping with myriad side effects. I'm also nervous about what the future will bring. I'm curious about how I will spend my time when it's not spent dealing with treatments and doctors' appointments. I'm cautious to move forward as a cancer survivor. I'm worried that the cancer will return. But through all these feelings, I keep coming back to the idea that living in the moment is all I truly have.

Now is the time to trust myself, to trust my instincts. To understand that yes, I was one of the many, many women diagnosed with breast cancer each year, but to also know that I am one of one, one of me. And it's time for me to trust myself enough to follow my own, unique path.

I feel as if I am standing on the edge of a seaside cliff—the sun on my face, feeling the sea breeze. I am looking out into the rest of my life. I'm a little nervous about that first step—will I be lifted into the wind, flying with arms open wide? Will I step forward to find a solid, bold path down the side of the cliff? The path is secondary. What is important, what is absolutely essential, is taking that first step into my new normal.

Life after zero treatments means...

Living in the moment because
I understand that this moment is all I have.

Knowing that each day is a blank page
And only I can decide what to put on it.

Accepting that there are no right or wrong choices,
There are only my choices.

Following my heart because
My heart knows the way.

Creating my new normal, my life,
With what is meaningful to me.

—Gayle Bittinger

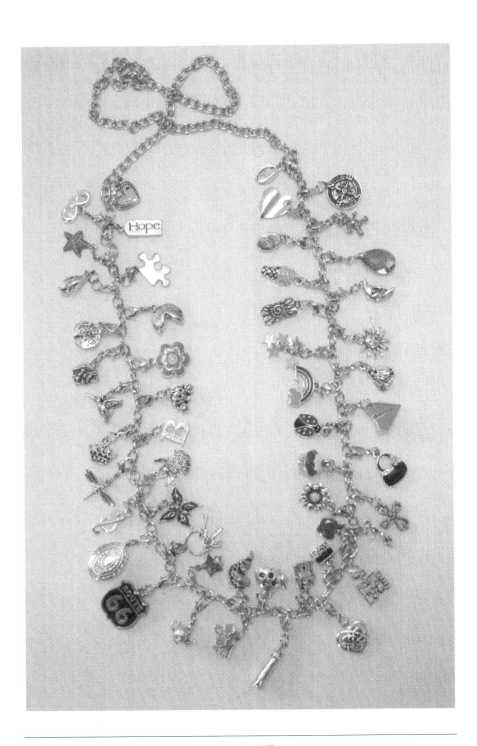

Breathe out worries
And breathe in peace of mind.

Breathe out anxiety
And breathe in calm.

Breathe out doubts
And breathe in joy.

Breathe out guilt
And breathe in gratitude.

Breathe out fear
And breathe in love.

—Gayle Bittinger

About the Author

Gayle Bittinger is a published author and editor of educational books and the Totline Magazine for preschool teachers. She has a B.A. in Family and Community Services from Western Washington University. Gayle lives in West Richland, Washington, with John, her husband of 30 years. Their daughter, Katie, is away doing graduate work, and their son, Alex, is in high school.

Gayle was diagnosed with a rare form of breast cancer in October 2010. She survived 18 months of aggressive treatments and enjoyed 15 months of living with no evidence of disease before being diagnosed with metastatic breast cancer in June 2013. Since her original diagnosis, Gayle and her family have made hundreds of sets of prayer beads to give away to cancer patients and their caregivers.

You can contact Gayle by email at sphereofhope@gmail.com.

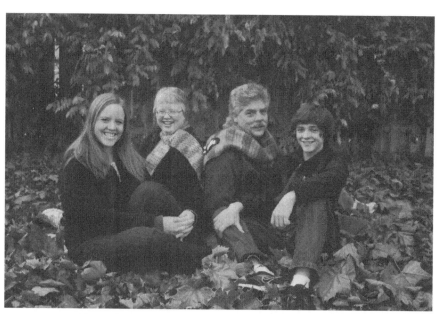

From right to left: Katie, Gayle, John, and Alex Bittinger

Made in the USA
San Bernardino, CA
03 September 2016